PENNSYLVANIA COLLEGE OF TECHNOLOGY LIB

D1111500

DAT

APR 2

Oral
Medicine

A Color Handbook of

Oral Medicine

RICHARD C.K. JORDAN DDS, MSc, PhD, FRCDC, Diplomate
Am B Oral & Max Pathology, Diplomate Am B Oral Medicine
Associate Professor of Oral Pathology and Pathology
University of California San Francisco, California

MICHAEL A.O. LEWIS PhD, BDS, FDSRCPS (Glas),
FDSRCS (Edin), FDSRCS (Eng), FRCPath
Professor of Oral Medicine
University of Wales College of Medicine, Cardiff, UK

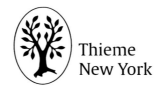

Thieme
New York

LIBRARY

JAN 0 9 2006

Pennsylvania College
of Technology

One College Avenue
Williamsport, PA 17701-5799

First published in the United States of America in 2004 by:
Thieme New York, 333 Seventh Avenue
New York, NY 10001, USA

ISBN 1–58890–274–9

Library of Congress Cataloging-in-Publication Data
is available from the publisher

This book, including all parts thereof, is legally protected by copyright. Any use, exploitation, or commercialization outside the narrow limits set by copyright legislation, without the publisher's consent, is illegal and liable to prosecution. This applies in particular to photostat reproduction, copying, mimeographing or duplication of any kind, translating, preparation of microfilms, and electronic data processing and storage.

Important note: Medical knowledge is ever-changing. As new research and clinical experience broaden our knowledge, changes in treatment and drug therapy may be required. The authors and editors of the material herein have consulted sources believed to be reliable in their efforts to provide information that is complete and in accord with the standards accepted at the time of publication. However, in view of the possibility of human error by the authors, editors, or publisher of the work herein, or changes in medical knowledge, neither the authors, editors, or publisher, nor any other party who has been involved in the preparation of this work, warrants that the information contained herein is in every respect accurate or complete, and they are not responsible for any errors or omissions or for the results obtained from use of such information. Readers are encouraged to confirm the information contained herein with other sources. For example, readers are advised to check the product information sheet included in the package of each drug they plan to administer to be certain that the information contained in this publication is accurate and that changes have not been made in the recommended dose or in the contraindications for administration. This recommendation is of particular importance in connection with new or infrequently used drugs.

Some of the product names, patents, and registered designs referred to in this book are in fact registered trademarks or proprietary names even though specific reference to this fact is not always made in the text. Therefore, the appearance of a name without designation as proprietary is not to be construed as a representation by the publisher that it is in the public domain.

Copyright © 2004 Manson Publishing Ltd, 73 Corringham Road, London NW11 7DL, UK

Commissioning editor: Jill Northcott
Project manager: Paul Bennett
Copy-editor: Kathryn Rhodes
Designer: Alpha Media
Color reproduction by Tenon & Polert Colour Scanning Ltd, Hong Kong
Printed in China by New Era Printing Company Ltd

Contents

LIBRARY

Preface

The primary aim of this book is to provide the clinician with a well-illustrated text that may be used firstly to assist the diagnosis of those conditions that fall into the specialty of oral medicine and secondly to provide a guide to initial treatment. A number of excellent atlas-type texts or reference works that comprehensively cover oral diseases are available. However, these books may be of limited value in the clinical setting since the material is usually presented according to the underlying etiology, such as infection, neoplasia, or developmental anomaly, rather than on the patient's symptomatic complaint of ulceration, erythema, white patch, or pain. It is hoped that the reader will find that the symptom-based approach employed in this book will be one of practical value in the clinical diagnosis and management of patients with oral diseases.

Richard C.K. Jordan
Michael A.O. Lewis

Acknowledgements

Professor Lewis is especially grateful to Heather for her love and understanding, not only during the writing of this book, but also in the past at the time of many other professional commitments. In addition, special recognition must go to Professor Derrick Chisholm, Professor of Dental Surgery, University of Dundee for his continual guidance and friendship throughout a period of twenty years.

Dr Jordan is grateful for the support and patience of his wife Yoon. He is also indebted to Dr Joseph Regezi of the University of California San Francisco for helpful discussions and advice. Special acknowledgement goes to Dr James Main at the University of Toronto for many years of education, mentoring, and friendship. In addition, he kindly provided some of the clinical illustrations for this book.

Both authors would like to acknowledge the help of Professor Bill Binnie, Baylor College of Dentistry, Dallas for his comments on the initial outline of this book. A particular thank you must also go to Jill Northcott, Commissioning Editor at Manson Publishing for her patience during the preparation and submission of the material of this book.

Clinical slides were also kindly provided by Dr Barbara Chadwick, Professor Graham Ogden, Mr Will McLaughlin, Mr Mike Cassidy, Professor Phil Lamey, Mr Mike Fardy, and Mr Andrew Cronin.

Abbreviations

ABH	Angina bullosa hemorrhagica	ITP	Idiopathic thrombocytopenia
ACE	Angiotensin-converting enzyme	KSHV	Kaposi's sarcoma herpesvirus
ACTH	Adrenocorticotropic hormone	LFTs	Liver function tests
AIDS	Acquired immune deficiency syndrome	MaRAS	Major recurrent aphthous stomatitis
ANUG	Acute necrotizing ulcerative gingivitis	MCV	Mean corpuscular volume
AZT	Azidothymidine	MiRAS	Minor recurrent aphthous stomatitis
BCG	Bacille Calmette–Guérin	MMP	Mucous membrane pemphigoid
BMS	Burning mouth syndrome	MRI	Magnetic resonance imaging
BMT	Bone marrow transplantation	MVD	Microvascular decompression
CREST	Subcutaneous calcinosis, Raynaud's phenomenon, esophageal dysfunction, sclerodactyly, and telangiectasia	PSA	Pleomorphic salivary adenoma
		PUVA	Psoralen and ultra-violet A
		RAS	Recurrent aphthous stomatitis
		RAS (HU)	Herpetiform recurrent aphthous stomatitis
CRP	C-reactive protein		
CT	Computerized tomography	RAST	Radio-allergen sorbent test
DLE	Discoid lupus erythematosis	REAL	Revised European American lymphoma
DNA	Deoxyribonucleic acid		
EBV	Epstein–Barr virus	SCC	Squamous cell carcinoma
ESR	Erythrocyte sedimentation rate	SLE	Systemic lupus erythematosis
FBC	Full blood count	SS	Sjögren's syndrome
FIGlu	Formimino glutamic acid	SSRI	Serotin re-uptake inhibitor
FTA abs	Fluorescent treponema/antibody absorbed	TENS	Transcutaneous electric nerve stimulation
GVHD	Graft versus host disease	TMJ	Temporomandibular joint dysfunction
HAD	Hospital Anxiety and Depression		
HHV	Human herpesvirus	TPHA	*Treponema pallidum* hemagglutination
HIV	Human immunodeficiency virus		
HLA	Human leukocyte antigen	VDRL	Venereal Diseases Reference Laboratory
HPV	Human papillomavirus		
HSV	Herpes simplex virus	VZV	Varicella zoster virus
IF	Immunofluorescence	WHO	World Health Organization

Chapter One

Introduction

- **A symptom-based approach to diagnosis**
- **History**
- **Clinical examination**
- **Normal structures**
- **Special investigation of orofacial disease**
- **Salivary gland investigations**

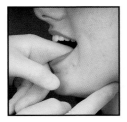
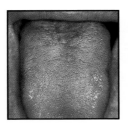
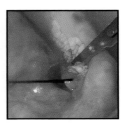
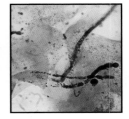

A symptom-based approach to diagnosis

A clinician's assessment of a patient presenting with a complaint of oral signs and symptoms may be viewed in a manner similar to that of a detective attempting to solve a crime. On some occasions the solution is straightforward, based on a short history obtained from the patient and examination of the lesion. On other occasions the diagnosis may be more elusive and require the analysis of a more complicated history and a more extensive clinical examination. In addition, special tests, in particular hematologic assessment, microbiologic sampling, and tissue biopsy, are of invaluable help in establishing the definitive diagnosis.

The material in this book has been grouped on the basis of the principal clinical sign or symptom obtained from the history and clinical examination.

History

A diagnosis can only be achieved after a detailed history of the complaint has been obtained. In addition, a full medical and dental history should be taken. Specific information related to the orofacial complaint should include details of site, onset, relieving and exacerbating factors. Further questioning often depends on the clinical signs observed but will usually include the following:

- First episode or recurrent problem? If recurrent, how many lesions and duration?
- Painful? If painful, nature, severity, timing, and duration?

Clinical examination

There is no 'right' or 'wrong' way to examine the orofacial tissues. However, it is essential to ensure that all areas and structures have been assessed in an organized and systematic fashion. Gloves should be worn throughout the examination.

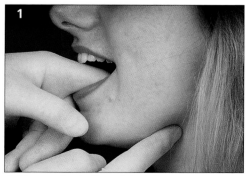

1 Bi-manual palpation of the left submandibular gland.

EXTRA-ORAL EXAMINATION
The clinical examination begins as soon as the patient presents in the clinic. Information on gait and the presence of any physical disability becomes evident as the patient gets into the examination chair. In the context of orofacial disease, the patient should be examined for obvious facial asymmetry and general appearance of the skin.

The lips should be examined for evidence of erythema and crusting, particularly at the angles. Any swelling within the lips should be palpated. The parotid gland should be palpated along with the cervical and neck lymph nodes. The sublingual and submandibular salivary glands should be palpated using a bi-manual technique (1). It may be necessary to assess function of each of the cranial nerves.

INTRA-ORAL EXAMINATION

A good light source and dental mirror are required for examination of the intra-oral structures. Initially an overall assessment should be made, although it likely that a more detailed examination of particular areas will be required later, depending on the signs and symptoms. The mucosa should appear moist and pink. Clear saliva should be present in the floor of the mouth.

The teeth should be examined for evidence of gross caries, discoloration, and presence of plaque or calculus. Any relationship between the teeth or restorations and mucosal abnormalities should be noted. The entire oral mucosa should be examined, including dorsum and lateral margins of the tongue, buccal and labial mucosa, hard and soft palate, and floor of the mouth (**2–8**).

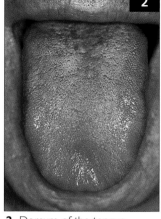

2 Dorsum of the tongue.

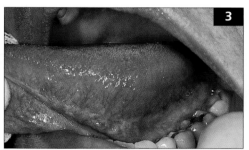

3 Left lateral margin of the tongue.

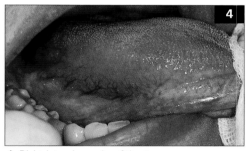

4 Right lateral margin of the tongue.

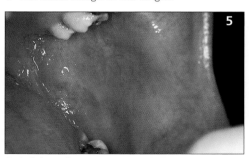

5 Left buccal mucosa.

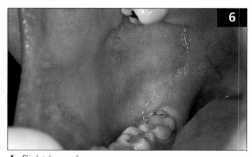

6 Right buccal mucosa.

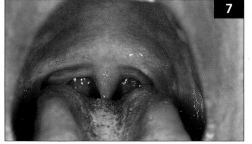

7 Soft and hard palate.

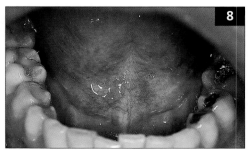

8 Floor of the mouth.

Normal structures

Normal structures within the mouth are sometimes mistaken for pathologic conditions. Examples of this are the circumvallate papillae (9) and foliate papillae (10) of the tongue, fissured tongue (11, 12), lingual varicosities (13), and ectopic sebaceous glands (14).

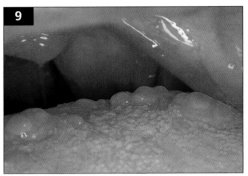

9 Circumvallate papillae at the junction of the anterior two-thirds and the posterior third of the tongue.

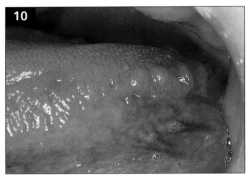

10 Foliate papillae on the posterior lateral margin of the tongue.

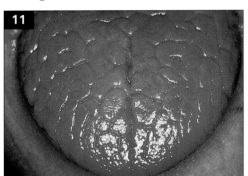

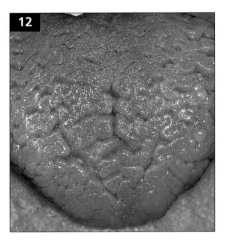

11, 12 Fissured tongue.

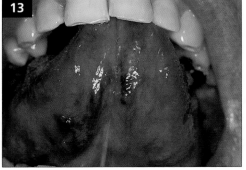

13 Lingual varicosities.

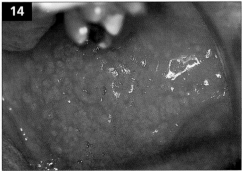

14 Ectopic sebaceous glands.

Special investigation of orofacial disease

The special investigations that are employed in oral medicine may be grouped under four headings: hematologic, microbiologic, tissue biopsy, and salivary gland investigations.

HEMATOLOGIC ASSESSMENT
The range of hematologic tests available to assist in diagnosis of oral facial disease is large. Details of specific tests required for each condition presented in this book are given within the main text.

MICROBIOLOGIC INVESTIGATION
Smear
A smear may be obtained by spreading material scraped from a lesion onto a glass microscope slide and examined for the presence of bacteria or fungi using Gram stain (**15**).

Plain swab
A plain microbiologic swab can be used to detect the presence of bacteria (**16**), fungi, herpes simplex viruses, or varicella zoster virus. Swabs should be sent to the laboratory promptly. Viral swabs should be placed in a transport medium (**17**).

IMPRINT CULTURE
An imprint culture may be used to determine bacteriologic or fungal colonization of the mucosa or surface of a denture or other intra-oral appliances. A foam square is held on the lesional site for 30 seconds prior to placement on a culture medium in the clinic. This method is site specific and provides a semi-quantitative assessment of colonization (**18**).

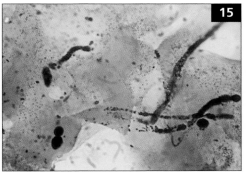

15 Smear from an angle of the mouth stained by Gram's method showing epithelial cells, candidal hyphae, and spores (blue).

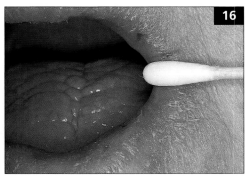

16 Swab of an angle of the mouth.

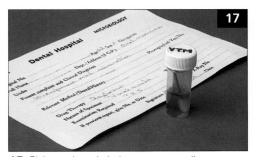

17 Plain swab and viral transport medium.

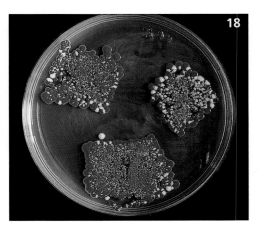

18 Imprint cultures on chromogenic agar showing a heavy mixed growth of *Candida albicans* (white) and *C. glabrata* (red).

CONCENTRATED ORAL RINSE

The concentrated oral rinse technique comprises 10 ml of phosphate buffered saline that is held in the mouth for 1 minute prior to re-collection (19). This method provides a semi-quantitative assessment of the overall oral microflora.

MUCOSAL BIOPSY

Mucosal biopsy can be performed under local anesthesia placed immediately adjacent to the lesional tissue (20). An ellipse of tissue that includes the periphery of the lesion is obtained using two incisions (21–27). Alternatively, a 5 mm dermatologic punch biopsy may be used to obtain a core of tissue suitable for histopathologic examination. The biopsy material should be supported on filter paper to prevent the specimen twisting or curling up when placed in formalin. Tissue for immunofluorescence studies should be sent to the laboratory fresh, on ice, or in Michel's medium.

EXFOLIATE CYTOLOGY AND BRUSH BIOPSY

Exfoliate cytology is a sampling method that involves the examination of cells obtained from the surface of mucosal lesions on a spatula and spread onto a glass microscope slide. Brush biopsy is a similar type of investigation but employs the application of a brush (28) to the lesion to collect a sample that includes not only superficial cells but also those from the basal layer. These techniques have been developed as a method of monitoring epithelial dysplasia and detecting squamous cell carcinoma. Both methods at the present time are problematic and further validation of their usefulness is required. However, if such investigation reveals any suggestion of atypical cells, then a biopsy is mandatory.

VITAL STAINING

Tolonium chloride (toluidine blue), a nuclear dye that has been used in the detection of carcinoma in the cervix of women, has also been applied to the mouth as an oral rinse. Abnormal areas of mucosa stain blue (29). However, extensive evaluation of tolonium chloride has not supported the technique as an accurate method for detection of oral dysplasia or carcinoma and its role is therefore questionable. The method may have a role as an adjunctive investigation to aid the selection of biopsy site in a patient with widespread mucosal lesions.

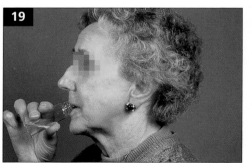

19 Method for concentrated oral rinse sampling of the oral flora.

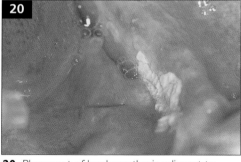

20 Placement of local anesthesia adjacent to the lesion.

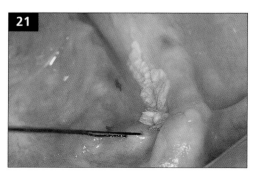

21 Suture placed anterior to the lesion.

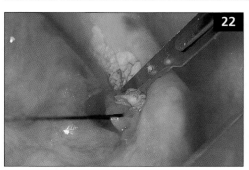

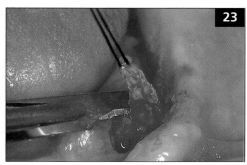

22, 23 An ellipse of tissue obtained using two incisions.

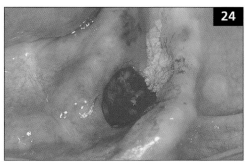

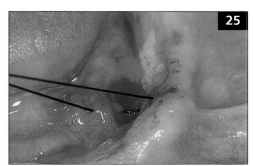

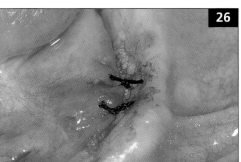

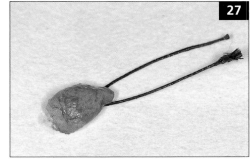

24–26 Wound closure using two single sutures.

27 Tissue supported on filter paper prior to placement in formal saline.

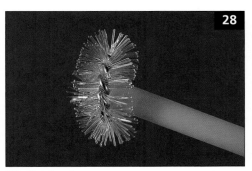

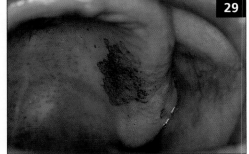

28 Cytobrush.

29 Blue-stained mucosa in the palate following topical application of tolonium chloride.

Salivary gland investigations

SALIVARY FLOW RATES
Mixed saliva flow can be measured either as simple collection of saliva at rest or following stimulation by chewing wax. Parotid gland flow can be assessed using a Carlsson–Crittenden cup (**30, 31**). Stimulation of the parotid gland can be achieved by placement of 1 ml of 10% citric acid on the dorsum of the tongue.

SIALOGRAPHY
Sialography involves the infusion of a radio-opaque dye, usually iodine-based, into a salivary gland through the submandibular or parotid duct (**32**). Radiographs will show the presence of any structural abnormality within the gland.

SCINTISCANNING
Scintiscanning involves the intravenous injection of a radio-active isotope, usually technetium (^{99M}TC) as pertechnetate. Uptake of the isotope within the head and neck is then measured using a gamma camera to visualize functional salivary tissue (**33**).

LABIAL GLAND BIOPSY
Labial gland biopsy should involve the recovery of five or more lobules of gland tissue (**34**). The minor glands should be taken from an area of the lower lip with apparently normal overlying mucosa, since inflammatory changes in superficial tissues may result in secondary non-specific changes in the salivary glands.

SCHIRMER'S TEST
Lacrimal flow can be measured by Schirmer's test which involves placement of a filter paper strip under the lower eyelid for 5 minutes (**35**). Wetting of the paper of less than 5 mm is indicative of reduced tear production.

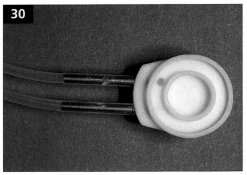

30 Carlson–Crittenden cup.

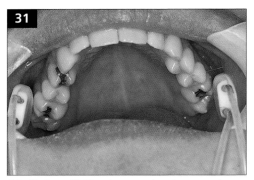

31 Carlson–Crittenden cup placed over each parotid papilla.

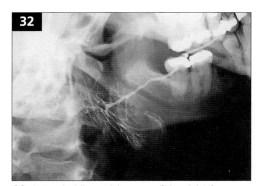

32 Lateral oblique sialogram of the right parotid gland showing the normal gland and duct architecture.

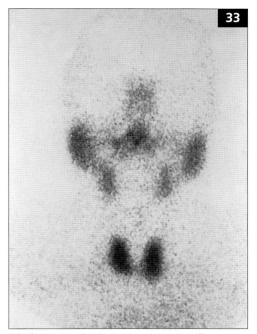

33 Scintiscan showing normal uptake of technetium in the thyroid glands and salivary tissues.

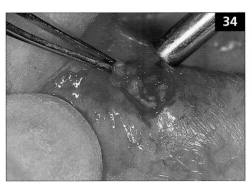

34 Labial gland biopsy.

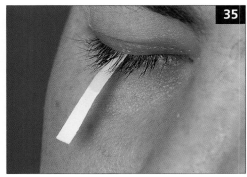

35 Schirmer's lacrimal flow test.

Ulceration

- **General approach**
- **Traumatic ulceration**
- **Recurrent aphthous stomatitis**
- **Behçet's disease**
- **Cyclic neutropenia**
- **Squamous cell carcinoma**
- **Necrotizing sialometaplasia**
- **Tuberculosis**
- **Syphilis**
- **Acute necrotizing ulcerative gingivitis**
- **Erosive lichen planus**
- **Lichenoid reaction**
- **Graft versus host disease**
- **Radiotherapy-induced mucositis**
- **Osteoradionecrosis**

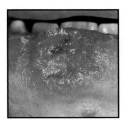
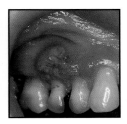
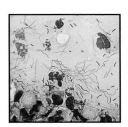
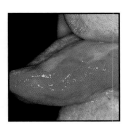

General approach

- Ulceration of the oral mucosa may be due to trauma, infection, immune-related disease, or neoplasia. Vesicullobullous blistering disorders frequently also present as ulceration due to rupture of initial lesions (Chapter 3, p. 42).
- Oral ulcers are invariably painful, although an important exception is squamous cell carcinoma, which is often painless, particularly when the tumor is small.
- Ulceration may represent neoplasia and therefore biopsy should be undertaken if there is any suspicion of malignancy or there is uncertainty of alternative diagnoses.
- Due to the good vascularity of the oral tissues the majority of ulcers in the mouth heal relatively quickly. Therefore, any ulcer persisting beyond 14 days should be considered neoplastic until proven otherwise.

Table 1 shows patterns of ulceration and likely diagnoses.

Table 1 Patterns of ulceration

Single or small number of discrete ulcers
- Traumatic ulceration
- Minor and major recurrent aphthous stomatitis
- Cyclic neutropenia
- Behçet's disease
- Squamous cell carcinoma
- Necrotizing sialometaplasia
- Tuberculosis
- Syphilis

Multiple discrete ulcers
- Herpetiform recurrent aphthous stomatitis
- Behçet's disease
- Acute necrotizing ulcerative gingivitis

Multiple diffuse ulceration
- Erosive lichen planus
- Lichenoid reaction
- Graft versus host disease
- Radiotherapy-induced mucositis
- Osteoradionecrosis

Traumatic ulceration

ETIOLOGY AND PATHOGENESIS
Traumatic causes of oral ulceration may be physical or chemical. Physical damage to the oral mucosa may be caused by sharp surfaces within the mouth, such as components of dentures, orthodontic appliances, dental restorations, or prominent tooth cusps. In addition, some patients suffer ulceration as a result of the irritation of cheek chewing. Oral ulceration caused during seizures is well-recognized in poorly-controlled epileptics. Chemical irritation of the oral mucosa may produce ulceration; a common cause is placement of aspirin tablets or caustic toothache remedies on the mucosa adjacent to painful teeth or under dentures. Situations also occasionally arise where a patient with psychologic problems may deliberately cause ulceration in their mouth (factitial ulcers).

CLINICAL FEATURES
Traumatic ulceration characteristically presents as a single localized deep ulcer (**36**, **37**) with, as would be expected from physical injury, an irregular outline. In contrast, chemical irritation may present as a more widespread superficial area of erosion, often with a slough of fibrinous exudate (**38**).

DIAGNOSIS
The cause of a traumatic lesion is often obvious from the history or clinical examination. Factitial ulceration is usually more difficult to diagnose since the patient may be less forthcoming with the history; therefore a high index of suspicion is necessary to establish the diagnosis. Biopsy is often needed to establish the diagnosis and to rule out infection or neoplasia.

MANAGEMENT

If traumatic ulceration is suspected and it is possible to eliminate the cause, such as smoothing of a tooth or repairing a denture or restoration, and if the mouth can be kept clean, healing will result within 7–10 days. If the lesion is particularly painful then the use of sodium bicarbonate in water or antiseptic mouthwashes, such as chlorhexidine or benzydamine, may be helpful. A biopsy, to exclude the presence of neoplasia such as carcinoma, lymphoma, or salivary gland tumor, should be taken from any ulcer that fails to heal within 2 weeks of the removal of the suspected cause. A patient who is thought to be deliberately self-inducing an ulcer may be challenged with this diagnosis, although admission by the patient is uncommon, and the underlying psychologic problems should be explored with appropriate specialist help.

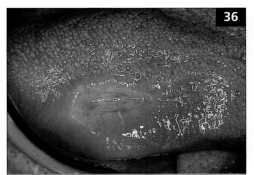

36 Ulcer on the lateral margin of the tongue induced by trauma from the edge of a fractured restoration in the first lower molar.

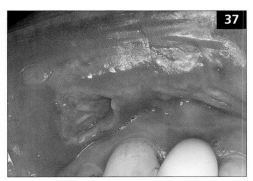

37 Irregular ulcer that was self-induced by the patient.

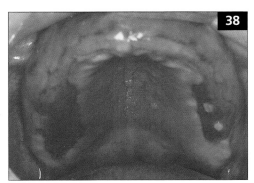

38 Diffuse ulceration in the palate due to the placement of salicyclic acid gel by the patient onto the fitting surface of her upper denture.

Recurrent aphthous stomatitis

ETIOLOGY AND PATHOGENESIS

In Western Europe and North America, recurrent aphthous stomatitis (RAS) is the most frequent mucosal disorder, affecting approximately 15–20% of the population at some time in their lives. Although many etiologic theories have been proposed for RAS, no single causative factor has as yet been identified. Hematinic deficiency involving reduced levels of iron, folic acid, or vitamin B_{12} has been found in a minority of patients with RAS and correction has led to resolution of symptoms. Other predisposing factors implicated include: psychologic stress, hypersensitivity to foodstuffs, cessation of smoking, and penetrative injury. However, in the majority of sufferers, it is difficult to identify a definite cause for their RAS.

CLINICAL FEATURES

Clinically, RAS may be divided into three subtypes: minor, major, and herpetiform. All types of RAS share common presenting features of regular, round or oval, painful ulcers with an erythematous border that recur on a regular basis.

The large majority of patients with RAS suffer from the minor form (MiRAS) characterized by either a single or a small number of shallow ulcers that are approximately 5 mm in diameter or less (**39, 40**). MiRAS affects the nonkeratinized sites within the mouth, such as the labial mucosa, buccal mucosa, or floor of the mouth. Keratinized mucosa is rarely involved and therefore MiRAS are not usually seen in the hard palate or on the attached gingivae. The ulcers of MiRAS typically heal in 10–14 days without scarring, if kept clean.

Major recurrent aphthous stomatitis (MaRAS) occurs in approximately 10% of patients with RAS and, as the name implies, the clinical features are more severe than those seen in the minor form. Ulcers, typically 1–3 cm in diameter (**41**), occur either singly or two or three at a time and usually last for 4–6 weeks. Any oral site may be affected, including keratinized sites. Clinical examination may reveal scarring of the mucosa at sites of previous lesions, due to the severity and prolonged nature of MaRAS.

Herpetiform RAS (HU) presents with ulcers similar to those of MiRAS but in this form the number of ulcers is increased and often involves as many as 50 separate lesions (**42**). The term 'herpetiform' has been used since the clinical presentation of HU may resemble primary herpetic gingivostomatitis, but at the present time members of the herpes group of viruses have not been found to be involved in this or in either of the other two forms of RAS.

DIAGNOSIS

Diagnosis of RAS is made relatively easily due to the characteristic clinical appearance of the ulcers and the recurrent nature of the symptoms. A biopsy may be necessary in some patients with MaRAS since a solitary lesion may resemble neoplasia or deep fungal infection.

MANAGEMENT

A wide range of treatment has been recommended for the symptomatic management of RAS. However, in addition to providing treatment to reduce pain and aid healing of lesions, it may be helpful to identify predisposing factors. All patients with RAS should be advised to avoid foods containing benzoate preservatives (E210–219), potato chips, crisps, and chocolate since many sufferers implicate these foods in the onset of ulcers. Any relationship to gastrointestinal disease, menstruation, and stress should be investigated. Hematologic deficiency should be excluded, particularly if the patient has gastrointestinal symptoms, heavy menstrual blood loss, or a vegetarian diet. Blood investigation should include a full blood count and assessment of vitamin B_{12}, corrected whole blood folate and ferritin levels. Patients may also relate the onset of ulceration to periods of psychologic stress.

Many patients obtain symptomatic relief from use of a mouthwash (sodium bicarbonate in water, chlorhexidine, or benzydamine) or application of topical corticosteroids preparations (hydrocortisone, triamcinolone, beclomethasone or betamethasone). A mouthwash based on tetracycline (250 mg capsule broken into water and used 4 times daily for 1 week) has also been found to be helpful.

Systemic immunomodulating drugs and other agents, such as prednisolone (prednisone), levamisole, monoamine oxidase inhibitors, thalidomide or dapsone, can successfully control RAS, but their use should be considered carefully and they are best prescribed in specialist units for patients who do not respond to topical therapy.

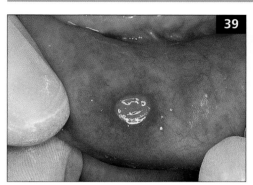

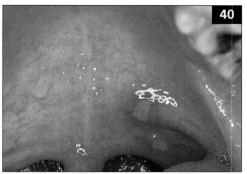

39 Small round ulcer (MiRAS) affecting the labial mucosa.

40 Small round and oval ulcers (MiRAS) affecting the soft palate.

41 Large round ulcer (MaRAS) in the buccal mucosa.

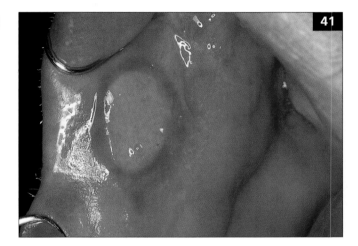

42 Multiple small round and oval ulcers (HU) in the soft palate.

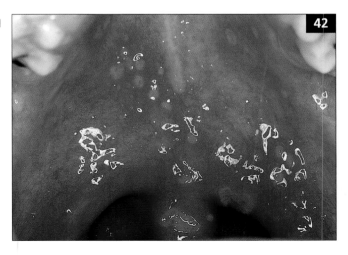

Behçet's disease

ETIOLOGY AND PATHOGENESIS

The etiology of Behçet's disease remains unclear but is known to involve aspects of the immune system. There is a strong association between Behçet's disease and the HLA B51 haplotype.

CLINICAL FEATURES

Behçet's disease is a multi-system condition with a range of manifestations including oral and genital ulceration, arthritis, cardiovascular disease, thrombophlebitis, cutaneous rashes, and neurologic disease. The condition usually begins in the third decade of life and is slightly more common in males than in females. Behçet's disease is more common in certain Mediterranean countries and in some Asian countries, especially Japan. The oral lesions consist of ulceration that may be any of the three forms of recurrent aphthous stomatitis, although the lesions tend to be of the major type (**43**), which heal with scarring (**44**).

DIAGNOSIS

Recurrent oral ulceration is an essential feature of Behçet's disease, but a number of other criteria are required to be fulfilled to establish the diagnosis. HLA typing may be of value.

MANAGEMENT

Oral lesions should be managed symptomatically in the same way as recurrent aphthous stomatitis. The systemic manifestations are managed by the patient's physician.

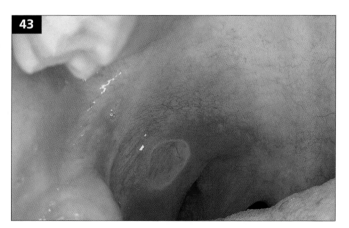

43 An ulcer of major aphthous stomatitis in the palate of a patient with Behçet's disease.

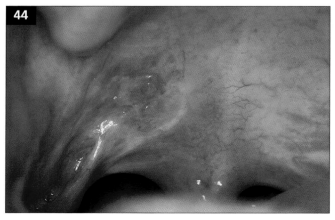

44 Scarring following the resolution of major aphthous stomatitis.

Cyclic neutropenia

ETIOLOGY AND PATHOGENESIS

Neutropenia is defined as an absolute reduction in circulating neutrophils. Prolonged or persistent neutropenia is associated with leukemia, some blood dyscrasias, many drugs, and radiation or chemotherapy. Cyclic neutropenia is a rare disorder of unknown etiology where there is a severe, cyclical depression of neutrophils from the blood and bone marrow.

CLINICAL FEATURES

During episodes of neutropenia there is fever, malaise, cervical lymphadenopathy, infections, and oral ulcers. Oral ulceration is common on nonkeratinized surfaces and may appear as single (**45, 46**) or multiple discrete lesions. Patients are also prone to severe periodontal disease.

DIAGNOSIS

Diagnosis is established on examination of the peripheral blood differential showing a reduction in circulating neutrophils during episodes of oral ulceration.

MANAGEMENT

There is no specific management for the condition. Medical investigations may be needed to rule out other causes of neutropenia. During episodes of neutropenia, antibiotics may be given to prevent oral infection. Scrupulous oral hygiene is needed to minimize periodontal disease.

45, 46 Minor aphthous stomatitis in cyclic neutropenia.

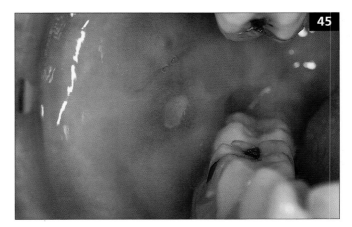

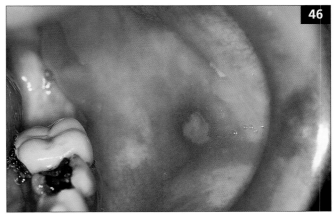

Squamous cell carcinoma

ETIOLOGY AND PATHOGENESIS

The vast majority of intra-oral malignancies are cases of squamous cell carcinoma (SCC). A number of etiologic factors have been proposed for SCC but at the present time the two most important are believed to be tobacco and alcohol. The smoking of tobacco in the form of cigarettes, cigars, or a pipe accounts for the majority of tobacco usage and there is a direct relationship between the amount of tobacco used and the risk of developing oral SCC. Although there has been some suggestion that smokeless tobacco is also associated with oral SCC, this link remains weak and controversial. By contrast, the chewing of 'pan soupari' (tobacco, areca nut, and slake lime) is a major cause of oral cancer in the Indian sub-continent.

Excessive drinking of alcohol is associated with an increased likelihood of occurrence of oral SCC. Interestingly, it has been observed that there is an adverse synergistic effect between tobacco and alcohol, with a greatly increased risk of SCC if a patient has both habits rather than just one. Other factors, such as deficiency of iron, vitamin A or vitamin C, fungal infection, viral infection, and stress have been proposed as being involved in the development of oral SCC, but their relative contributions and significance are unknown. While trauma itself would not appear to cause cancer, it has been implicated as a cofactor in the presence of another factor.

CLINICAL FEATURES

The clinical presentation of SCC can vary greatly and range from a small erythematous patch through to a large swelling or area of ulceration. SCC of the lip usually presents as a painless ulcer with rolled margins (**47**) and is associated with sun damage to the tissues. The majority of cases of SCC within the mouth develop in a previously clinical normal mucosa, although some may be preceded by a leukoplakia or an erythroplakia (Chapters 4, p. 74, and 5, p. 93). Approximately 70% of oral SCC develop in the floor of the mouth (**48**), tongue (**49**, **50**), or retromolar region (**51**). Although the gingivae are rarely affected, painless areas of ulceration at this site should be regarded as suspicious (**52**). Unfortunately, SCC is often painless at an early stage and therefore most (60–70%) of patients present with advanced (late stage) lesions involving metastatic spread to regional lymph nodes.

DIAGNOSIS

Although there are presenting features, such as induration and rolled margins, that may suggest the presence of oral SCC, the disease *cannot* be diagnosed clinically. Biopsy and histologic examination of lesion material is mandatory. The use of exfoliative cytology, topical nuclear dye (tolinium chloride), and brush biopsy have all been suggested as a method for investigating suspicious mucosal lesions, but the usefulness of these techniques is uncertain and limited at the present time.

MANAGEMENT

Overall, the 5-year survival rate from oral cancer is approximately 40%, although this varies according to site. Lip cancer has the best 5-year survival rate of 90%, possibly due to the increased likelihood of detection of the tumor while small and the ease of treatment. By contrast, SCC of the floor of the mouth carries a poor prognosis, with a 5-year survival rate of around 20%. The most important predictor of outcome is the stage of the disease at presentation. The presence of metastatic tumor within the lymph node of the neck reduces the overall survival rate of oral SCC from any intra-oral site by 50%.

The treatment of oral cancer consists primarily of surgery, radiotherapy, or a combination of both approaches. Some patients may also receive chemotherapy prior (neo-adjuvant), during (concurrent), or after (adjuvant) treatment with radiotherapy. The development of microvascular surgery and use of free flaps in reconstruction has dramatically improved the quality of life for patients with SCC. Unfortunately, despite these surgical advances the post-operative survival rate of patients has changed little in the past 80 years, due to death from new primary lesions or metastases.

All patients with a history of SCC should be kept on long-term review to detect any recurrence of tumor or the development of further primary lesions. Obviously, patients should be given support to eliminate any tobacco and alcohol habit. Since outcome is influenced by early detection, all health care workers should regularly undertake examination of the oral mucosa of their patients. Dental surgeons are ideally placed to carry out this examination and represent one category of the key workers who could possibly improve the early detection of oral cancer. Any suspicious area of mucosa such as a persistent area of ulceration, leukoplakia, or erythroplakia should be biopsied. This could be carried out in the general dental practice setting but in cases of widespread mucosal involvement it may be more sensible to refer the patient to a specialist clinic.

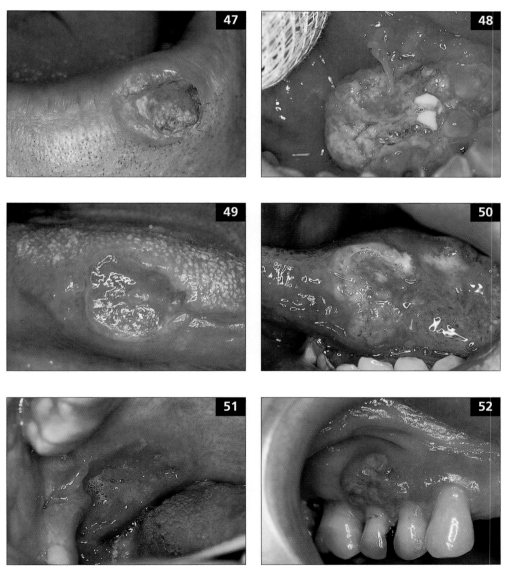

47–52 Squamous cell carcinoma presenting as an ulcer with rolled indurated margins on the lip and at a variety of intra-oral sites.

Necrotizing sialometaplasia

ETIOLOGY AND PATHOGENESIS
This is a benign salivary condition that occurs almost exclusively in the hard palate, although other sites where minor salivary glands are located may be affected. The condition is caused by local ischemia secondary to altered local blood supply, which in turn causes infarction of the salivary glands. Local trauma through injury or surgical manipulation is believed to be the most important etiologic factor.

CLINICAL FEATURES
Necrotizing sialometaplasia is characterized by the development of a painless swelling with dusky erythema in the hard palate, which ulcerates (**53**). Interestingly, there is often an associated anesthesia in the affected area. The clinical presentation can resemble squamous cell carcinoma (**54**), although the latter is relatively rare on the hard palate. A solitary lesion is usual but bilateral cases have occasionally been reported.

DIAGNOSIS
A biopsy is required to make the diagnosis. Specialist interpretation is essential since cases of necrotizing sialometaplasia have been falsely diagnosed histopathologically as squamous cell carcinoma.

MANAGEMENT
The condition is benign and self-limiting. An antiseptic mouthwash or spray should be used to treat the ulceration. Healing will occur within 6–10 weeks. Recurrence is unusual and there is no functional impairment.

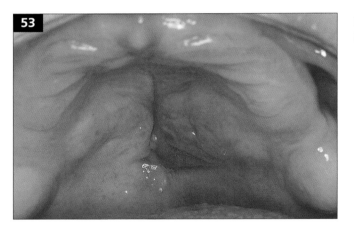

53 Necrotizing sialometaplasia presents initially as a swelling.

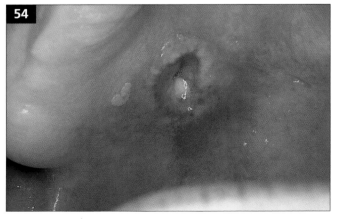

54 Subsequent ulceration in necrotizing sialometaplasia.

Tuberculosis

ETIOLOGY AND PATHOGENESIS
Tuberculosis is one of the most prevalent infectious diseases in the world, particularly in developing countries. Although tuberculosis is considered to be relatively rare in Western countries, it is being reported more frequently in recent years due to migration patterns from the developing to the developed world and the spread of HIV. Infection is spread in droplets of sputum containing the acid-fast bacillus, *Mycobacterium tuberculosis,* from patients with active pulmonary tuberculosis. In some patients infection also produces lesions within the oral cavity.

CLINICAL FEATURES
The classical intra-oral presentation is of an ulcer on the dorsal surface of the tongue but lesions may affect any site (**55**). The ulcers are irregular with raised borders and may resemble deep fungal infection or squamous cell carcinoma.

DIAGNOSIS
Mucosal biopsy should be undertaken to demonstrate characteristic granulomatous inflammation with well-formed granulomata, Langhan's giant cells, and necrosis. Ziehl–Neelsen or Fite stains may be used to detect tubercle bacilli. Microbiologic culture of suspected clinical material may also be useful to establish the diagnosis of tuberculosis. It is important to inform the microbiologist that tuberculosis is suspected because specialized media (Lowenstein–Jensen's) and prolonged incubation (2–3 months) is required for recovery of the organism. Molecular microbiologic methods are being used increasingly to establish the diagnosis. A Mantoux (tuberculin) skin test will be positive as a result of previous infection in patients who have not received prior BCG immunization. Previous infection may occasionally be seen as incidental radio-opacities on radiographs due to calcification within lymph nodes (**56**).

MANAGEMENT
Localized treatment is not required because oral lesions will resolve when systemic chemotherapy with rifampin (rifampicin), isoniazid, or ethambutol is administered. Typically, combinations of these drugs are used for 9 months–2 years of treatment. Worryingly, strains of *M. tuberculosis* that are resistant to many of the drugs that have traditionally been used to treat this infection are being encountered. In the future there may be difficulty in treating this condition.

55 Tuberculous ulcer on the tongue.

56 Radiograph showing a radio-opaque mass due to tuberculosis within the submandibular lymph nodes.

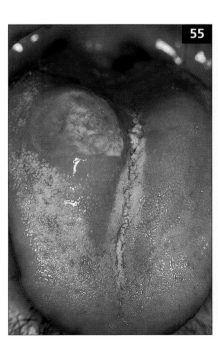

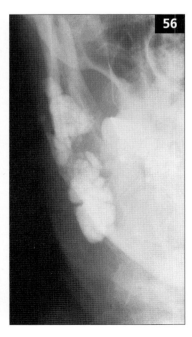

Syphilis

ETIOLOGY AND PATHOGENESIS
Syphilis is caused by the spirochete *Treponema pallidum*. Although the primary lesion of this sexually-transmitted disease usually occurs on the genitals, it may also present on the lips or oral mucosa as a result of orogenital contact.

CLINICAL FEATURES
Syphilis occurs in three stages: primary, secondary, and tertiary forms. The primary lesion, chancre, is characterized by the development of a firm nodule at the site of innoculation, which breaks down after a few days to leave a painless ulcer with indurated margins (**57**). Cervical lymph nodes are usually enlarged and rubbery in consistency. The chancre is highly infectious and therefore should be examined with caution. The lesions of primary syphilis usually resolve within 3–12 weeks without scarring.

Secondary syphilis appears clinically approximately 6 weeks or longer after the primary infection and is characterized by a macular or papular rash, febrile illness, malaise, headache, generalized lymphadenopathy, and sore throat. The oral mucosa is involved in approximately one-third of patients. Oral ulceration (**58**), described as 'snail track ulcers', develops. Lesions of secondary syphilis are infective but resolve within 2–6 weeks.

Approximately 30% of patients with untreated secondary syphilis develop the latent form many years after the initial infection. Fortunately, lesions of tertiary syphilis are now rarely seen in the West due to the successful treatment of the earlier stages. Two oral lesions are recognized in the tertiary form of syphilis: gumma in the palate and leukoplakia affecting the dorsal surface of the tongue.

A pregnant patient with primary or secondary syphilis may infect the developing fetus, resulting in characteristic congenital abnormalities (congenital syphilis). Infection of the developing vomer produces a nasal deformity known as saddle nose. The features of Hutchinson's triad include interstitial keratitis, deafness, and dental abnormalities consisting of notched or screwdriver-shaped incisors (**59**) and mulberry molars (**60**).

DIAGNOSIS
Diagnosis is supported if dark-field microscopy of a smear taken from either a primary or a secondary lesion reveals numerous spirochetes in size and form typical of *T. pallidum*. However, serologic investigation (10 ml clotted sample) is the most reliable way of diagnosing syphilis from the late stage of primary infection onwards, because *T. pallidum* cannot be routinely cultured *in vitro*. Venereal Diseases Reference Laboratory (VDRL), *T. pallidum* hemagglutination (TPHA), and fluorescent treponema/antibody absorbed (FTA abs) tests should be undertaken.

MANAGEMENT
The most effective treatment of any stage of syphilis is intramuscular procaine penicillin. *T. pallidum* has remained sensitive to penicillin, erythromycin, and tetracyclines. Patients should be followed up for at least 2 years and serologic examinations repeated over this period.

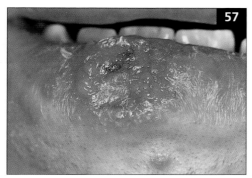

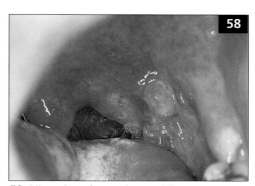

57 Ulcerated nodular lesion of primary syphilis.

58 Ulceration of secondary syphilis.

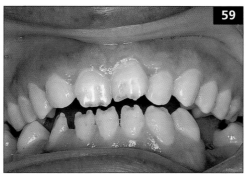

59 Notch deformity of the incisors due to congenital syphilis (Hutchinson's incisors).

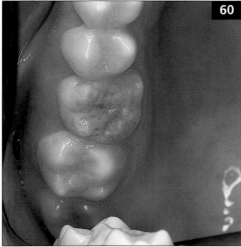

60 Hypoplastic deformity of the first molar due to congenital syphilis (Moon's molar, mulberry molar).

Acute necrotizing ulcerative gingivitis

ETIOLOGY AND PATHOGENESIS

The etiology of acute necrotizing ulcerative gingivitis (ANUG) is not fully understood but strictly anerobic bacteria, in particular spirochetes and *Fusobacterium* species, are likely to be involved since high numbers of these micro-organisms can be demonstrated in lesions. Furthermore, tobacco smoking and stress have been implicated as predisposing factors.

CLINICAL FEATURES

The classical presentation of ANUG comprises rapid development of painful ulceration affecting the gingival margin and inter-dental papillae (**61**, **62**) and is associated with a marked halitosis. The condition is usually widespread, although it may be limited to localized areas, the lower anterior region being most frequently affected.

DIAGNOSIS

The clinical history and symptoms are often sufficiently characteristic to permit diagnosis. If there is uncertainty, ANUG can be confirmed rapidly by microscopic examination of a Gram-stained smear taken from an area of ulceration that will show numerous fusobacteria, medium-sized spirochetes, and acute inflammatory cells (**63**).

MANAGEMENT

Initial management should involve thorough mechanical cleaning and debridement of the teeth in the affected area. In the past the use of hydrogen peroxide mouthwashes, both to provide mechanical cleansing and also to serve as an oxidizing agent, has been recommended, although the benefit of such treatment is not universally accepted. The importance of local measures cannot be over-emphasized, but symptoms will improve more rapidly if the patient is also given a systemic antimicrobial agent. Metronidazole (**200** mg 8-hourly) prescribed for 3 days will usually produce a dramatic improvement within 48 hours. In the long term, hygiene therapy to prevent further gingival damage should be arranged.

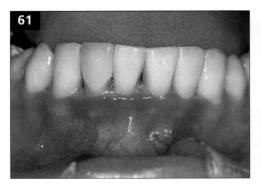

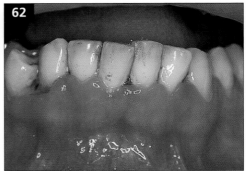

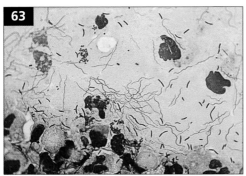

61, 62 Gingival ulceration and loss of the inter-dental papillae in the lower incisor region.

63 Smear from ANUG stained by Gram's method showing large numbers of fusiform bacteria and spirochetes.

Erosive lichen planus

ETIOLOGY AND PATHOGENESIS

Lichen planus is one of the more prevalent mucocutaneous disorders. The cause of lichen planus is not known, although it is immunologically mediated and resembles in many ways a hypersensitivity reaction to an unknown antigen. T-lymphocyte-mediated destruction of basal keratinocytes and hyperkeratinization produces the characteristic clinical lesions.

CLINICAL FEATURES

Lichen planus characteristically presents as white patches or striae that may affect any oral site (see Chapter 4). However, the clinical appearance is variable and the erosive form of the condition may produce oral ulceration (**64–66**).

DIAGNOSIS

Clinical diagnosis of oral lichen planus is aided by the presence of cutaneous lesions. If the main presenting feature is ulceration, further examination is likely to reveal areas of white patch or striae at other oral mucosa sites.

MANAGEMENT

The first line of treatment in symptomatic cases should consist of an antiseptic mouthwash combined with topical steroid therapy in the form of either hydrocortisone hemisuccinate pellets (2.5 mg) or betamethasone sodium phosphate (0.5 mg) allowed to dissolve on the affected area 2–4 times daily. Other preparations of topical steroid therapy, such as sprays, mouthwashes, creams, and ointments have been found to be beneficial for some patients. Intra-lesional injections of triamcinolone have also been tried with variable success. A short course of systemic steroid therapy may be required to alleviate acute symptoms in cases involving widespread ulceration, erythema, and pain. Other drugs used in lichen planus include ciclosporin (cyclosporin) mouthwash, topical tacrolimus, and systemic mycophenolate (Chapter 4, p. 60).

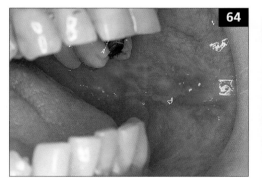

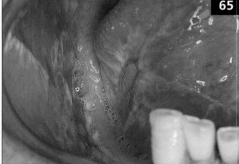

64–66 Erosive lichen planus presenting as ulceration in the buccal mucosa and floor of mouth.

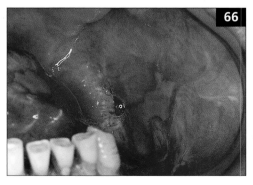

Lichenoid reaction

ETIOLOGY AND PATHOGENESIS
Lichenoid reactions are so-named because of the similarity, both clinically and histologically, to lichen planus. Systemic drugs, especially anti-hypertensives, hypoglycemics, and non-steroid anti-inflammatory agents, have been implicated in lichenoid drug reactions.

CLINICAL FEATURES
Although the clinical presentation of lichenoid reactions is characteristically seen as widespread irregular white patches (Chapter 4, p. 64), on occasions the mucosa may be extensively ulcerated (**67**) with sloughing (**68, 69**).

DIAGNOSIS
If oral lesions develop within a few weeks of the institution of drug therapy then there is likely to be a connection. Mucosal biopsy is not that helpful in supporting the diagnosis since the features are difficult to differentiate from lichen planus or may be non-specific.

MANAGEMENT
If the patient is taking a medicine known to be associated with the occurrence of lichenoid lesions, consideration should be given to a change of therapy to a structurally unrelated drug with similar therapeutic effect. Resolution of the mucosal lesions usually follows within a few weeks (Chapter 4, p. 64).

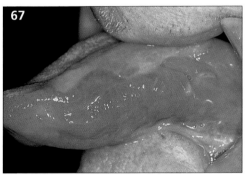

67 Ulceration caused by a lichenoid reaction to an anti-hypertensive drug.

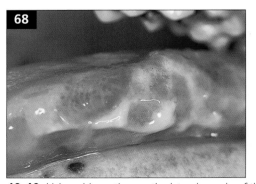

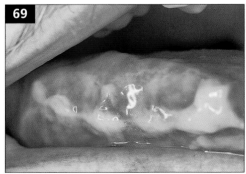

68, 69 Lichenoid reaction on the lateral margin of the tongue following systemic chemotherapy.

Graft versus host disease

ETIOLOGY AND PATHOGENESIS

Graft versus host disease (GVHD) occurs in patients who have received allogenic bone marrow transplantation (BMT). These patients will typically have had some form of major blood or bone marrow abnormality, such as leukemia, aplastic anemia, or widely disseminated malignancy. These conditions are treated with high-dose radiation and cytotoxic chemotherapy that result in destruction of normal hematopoetic cells. An HLA-matched bone marrow donor is then located and normal hematopoetic cells are transfused into the recipient. If the HLA matching is not exact then the engrafted lymphocytes target host cells, resulting in GVHD.

CLINICAL FEATURES

GVHD develops in acute and chronic forms related to the time of occurrence. Acute GVHD occurs in the next 100 days following allogenic BMT. Approximately 50% of all BMT recipients will develop acute GVHD. Manifestations range from various skin rashes and blisters to gastrointestinal symptoms such as vomiting, diarrhea, and liver dysfunction.

Chronic GVHD occurs during the next 100 days following BMT and mimics forms of auto-immune disease. Within the mouth there are white reticulated lesions that resemble erosive oral lichen planus (**70, 71**). Patients also often complain of burning of the mucosa secondary to candidosis (candidiasis) and xerostomia.

DIAGNOSIS

Diagnosis is challenging, particularly in the chronic stages of the disease, which may resemble other diseases both clinically and microscopically. A clinical history of BMT coupled with oral lesions may lead one to suspect GVHD; however, biopsy material is frequently nonspecific or may resemble lichen planus or lupus erythematosus.

MANAGEMENT

The most important management strategy is prevention. Careful HLA matching of BMT donor and recipient is important. Modulation of the immune response in the recipient is necessary, using immunosuppressive medications such as ciclosporin (cyclosporin). Psoralen and ultra-violet A (PUVA) therapy is helpful for cutaneous lesions. Suspected candidosis (candidiasis) needs to be confirmed microbiologically and treated appropriately. Xerostomia is managed symptomatically with salivary substitutes and burning can be relieved using topical anesthetic agents.

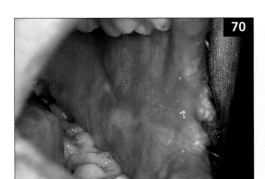 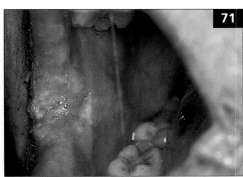

70, 71 Graft versus host disease presenting as diffuse erosion of the buccal mucosa.

Radiotherapy-induced mucositis

ETIOLOGY AND PATHOGENESIS
Patients who receive radiotherapy to the head and neck, as part of the treatment of malignancy, invariably develop a widespread and painful oral mucosal erosion or ulceration. Radiotherapy damages mitotic epithelial cells leading to epithelial breakdown, atrophy, ulceration, and inflammation. Superinfection by candida and staphylococci may also play a role in the development of radiation-induced mucositis.

CLINICAL FEATURES
The symptoms typically begin 1–2 weeks after the commencement of radiation therapy. There is a generalized erythema of the mucosa with areas of shallow ulceration and fibrinous exudate (72). Other features include pain, xerostomia, and loss of taste.

DIAGNOSIS
Diagnosis is usually straightforward due to the known history of radiotherapy that encompassed the orofacial tissues.

MANAGEMENT
Almost all patients receiving radiation therapy will develop stomatitis of varying severity. Generally, the condition will improve once radiation therapy is completed. During treatment, it is important that the patient keeps the mouth clean using a bland mouthwash such as sodium bicarbonate in water. Antibiotic and antifungal mouthwashes are also frequently used, although whether they provide any superior benefit compared to bland mouthwashes is not clear.

Osteoradionecrosis

ETIOLOGY AND PATHOGENESIS
Radiation is given to patients with many types of malignancy. When the treatment field encompasses the mandible and maxilla, there is the potential for osteoradionecrosis. Radiation affects the capacity of osteocytes, osteoblasts, and endothelial cells to repair following injury. Extraction of a tooth, peridodontal disease, and periapical infection are all factors that can predispose to the onset of osteoradionecrosis.

CLINICAL FEATURES
Osteoradionecrosis typically begins following minor trauma to the jaws. There is often ulceration and necrosis of the soft tissues, leaving areas of exposed bone. Small areas of necrosis, typically in the mandible, become larger and portions of necrotic bone are then lost (73, 74). The degree of osteoradionecrosis is usually proportional to the amount of radiation given. Traumatic tooth extraction is a common initiating factor for osteoradionecrosis. Other factors include poor oral hygiene, poor nutrition, and excess alcohol ingestion.

DIAGNOSIS
Diagnosis is established by history and clinical examination. Biopsy of the affected area will show necrotic tissues only and sequestration of bone.

MANAGEMENT
Prevention is by far the most important management strategy. Patients due to undergo radiotherapy in the region of the orofacial tissues should have a dental assessment prior to commencement of treatment. Any teeth with large or poor restorations, periapical infection, or periodontal disease should be extracted. Patients must have custom-made soft rubber dental trays fabricated for the delivery of topical neutral fluoride nightly.

Any extraction that is necessary following radiation therapy should be done in an atraumatic manner under antibiotic cover. Once osteoradionecrosis develops it is extremely difficult to treat, despite removal of necrotic bone and debridement. High-dose long-term antibiotic therapy is necessary. Hyperbaric oxygen treatments may also be helpful in order to increase oxgenation of the affected tissues.

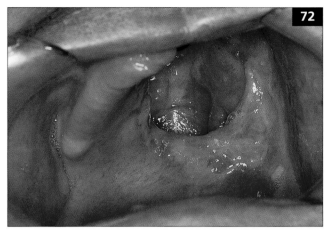

72 Mucositis following adjunctive radiotherapy and hemi-maxillectomy.

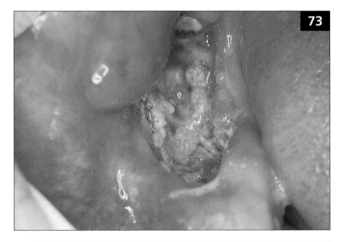

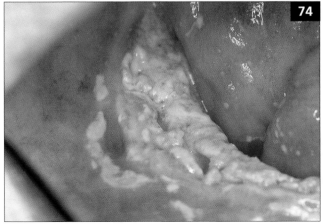

73, 74 Osteoradionecrosis.

Blisters

- **General approach**
- **Primary herpetic gingivostomatitis**
- **Recurrent herpes simplex infection**
- **Chickenpox and shingles**
- **Hand, foot, and mouth disease**
- **Herpangina**
- **Epidermolysis bullosa**
- **Mucocele**
- **Erythema multiforme**
- **Mucous membrane pemphigoid**
- **Pemphigus**
- **Linear IgA disease**
- **Dermatitis herpetiformis**
- **Angina bullosa hemorrhagica**

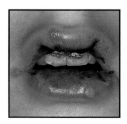
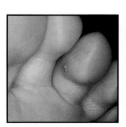
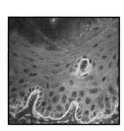
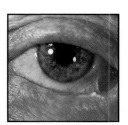

General approach

- Blistering of the oral mucosa may due to trauma, infection or immune-related disease. Although blistering disorders frequently affect the oral mucosa, it is rare to see intact vesicles or bullae since they rapidly rupture, leaving an area of erosion or ulceration (Chapter 2, p. 22).
- Blistering conditions are usually painful.
- The diagnosis of blistering disease invariably requires the use of immunofluorescence on biopsy material and serum. An important exception is herpetic infections.

Although blistering disease may develop at any age, the conditions may be divided into those occurring in younger individuals and those seen most frequently in adults or the elderly (*Table 2*).

Table 2 Patterns of blistering

Blistering conditions in children or young adults
- Primary herpetic gingivostomatitis
- Recurrent herpes simplex infection – labialis
- Recurrent herpes simplex infection – oral ulceration
- Chickenpox
- Hand, foot, and mouth disease
- Herpangina
- Mucocele

Blistering conditions in adulthood or the eldery
- Shingles
- Erythema multiforme
- Pemphigoid
- Pemphigus
- Linear IgA disease
- Dermatitis herpetiformis
- Angina bullosa hemorrhagica

Primary herpetic gingivostomatitis

ETIOLOGY AND PATHOGENESIS

This condition has been exclusively attributed to infection with herpes simplex virus (HSV) type I, although it is now recognized that HSV type II, traditionally associated with genital herpes, may occasionally be involved. Primary herpetic gingivostomatitis is the most frequent viral infection of the mouth and spreads easily through saliva. The source of infection may be an individual who is asymptomatically shedding virus in saliva or suffering a recurrent infection, such as herpes labialis. Herpes simplex virus initially infects the nonkeratinized epithelial cells of the oral mucosa to produce intra-epithelial blisters. Following recovery from primary infection, HSV resides latent in neural and other orofacial tissues. Examination of antibody status has revealed that more than 60% of the population of Europe and North America have evidence of HSV infection by the age of 16 years.

CLINICAL FEATURES

Primary infection often goes unnoticed or is dismissed as an episode of teething during childhood. However, it has been estimated that approximately 5% of individuals who first encounter the virus develop significant symptoms. The blisters of primary herpetic gingivostomatitis rupture rapidly to produce blood-crusted lips (**75, 76**) and widespread painful oral ulceration (**77, 78**). In addition, the gingivae are swollen and erythematous (**79**). The condition is associated with pyrexia, headache, and cervical lymphadenopathy.

DIAGNOSIS

Isolation and culture of HSV using a viral swab is the standard method of diagnosis. Confirmation of HSV infection can also be made serologically by the demonstration of a fourfold rise in antibody titer in acute and convalescent samples. Both these methods may take 10 days to provide a result. Chair-side kits that can rapidly detect within minutes the presence of HSV in a lesional smear using immunofluorescence are available, but their routine use is limited by cost. Biopsy is rarely necessary but if undertaken will show non-specific vesculation or ulceration with multinucleated giant cells representing viral-infected keratinocytes.

MANAGEMENT

Patients, and in the case of children usually their parents, should be reassured about the basis of the condition and advised of the infectious nature of the lesions. Instructions should be given to limit contact with the lips and mouth to reduce the risk of the spread of infection to other sites. Supportive symptomatic therapy should include a chlorhexidine mouthwash, analgesic therapy, soft diet, and adequate fluid intake. Use of aciclovir (acyclovir), an antiviral agent with activity against HSV, should be considered in severe cases. The standard regime is 200 mg aciclovir (acyclovir), either as a dispersible tablet or suspension 5 times daily for 5 days. The dosage should be halved in children under the age of 2 years.

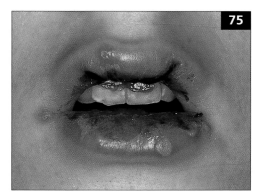

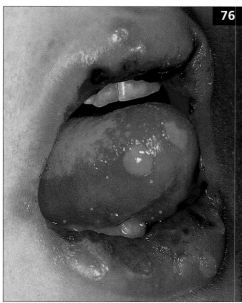

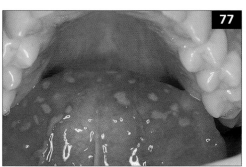

75–77 Vesicles, blood-crusting of the lips and multiple intra-oral ulcers characteristic of primary HSV infection.

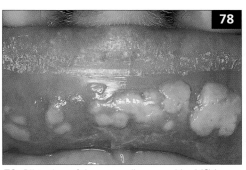

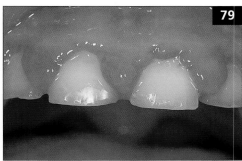

78 Blistering of the upper lip caused by HSV.

79 Swelling of the inter-dental papillae and gingival margins caused by HSV.

Recurrent herpes simplex infection

ETIOLOGY AND PATHOGENESIS

Secondary infection is caused by reactivation of latent HSV. Traditionally, it has been thought that HSV migrates from the trigeminal ganglion to the peripheral tissues. While this is possible it is becoming increasingly apparent that HSV also resides more locally in neural and other tissues. Up to 40% of HSV-positive individuals suffer from recurrent infections. The development of recurrent disease is related to either a breakdown in local immunosurveillance or an alteration in local inflammatory mediators that permits the virus to replicate.

CLINICAL FEATURES

Reactivation of HSV characteristically produces herpes labialis (cold sore, fever, blister). The symptoms of herpes labialis usually begin as a tingle or burning sensation (prodrome) in a localized region of the lips at the vermillion border. However, approximately 25% of episodes have no prodrome and the lesion presents directly as vesicles. Within 48 hours the vesicles rupture to leave an erosion which subsequently crusts over and eventually heals within 7–10 days (**80, 81**). Factors that predispose to the development of herpes labialis in susceptible individuals include sunlight, trauma, stress, fever, menstruation, and immunosuppression.

Reactivation of HSV can also produce recurrent intra-oral ulceration. Similar to herpes labialis, the patient with an intra-oral lesion is usually aware of prodromal tingling. The mucosa of the hard palate is the site most frequently involved (**82, 83**) but other areas such as the lower buccal sulcus or gingival margins (**84**) can also be affected. It can be difficult to determine whether the lesion(s) were precipitated by trauma in these patients or whether they chronically shed HSV in their saliva which subsequently colonizes traumatized mucosa.

DIAGNOSIS

The clinical appearance is usually diagnostic. Confirmation of the presence of HSV can be made by isolation from a swab in tissue culture or the use of immunofluorescence on a smear of a recent lesion.

MANAGEMENT

In many cases no active treatment is indicated but the patient should be warned about the infectivity of the lesion. The use of topical aciclovir (acyclovir) or penciclovir as early as possible can reduce the duration of herpes labialis. A sunscreen applied to the lips can also be effective in reducing the frequency of sunlight-induced recurrences.

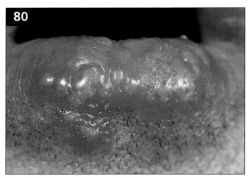

80 Vesicles of herpes labialis.

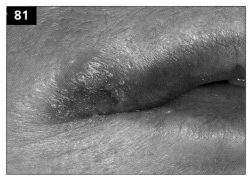

81 Crusting of a healing herpes labialis.

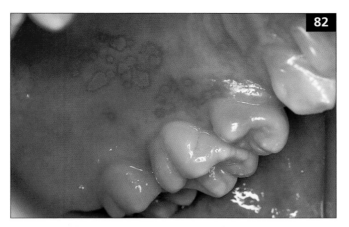

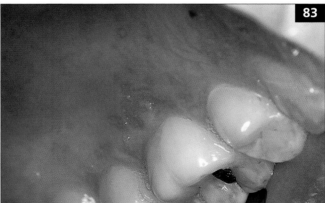

82, 83 Multiple ulcers in the hard palate, a frequent site of recurrent HSV infection.

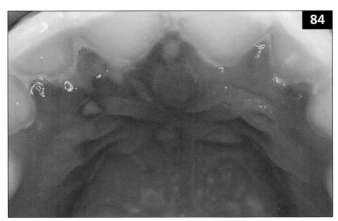

84 Ulceration of the gingival margins due to recurrent herpetic infection.

Chickenpox and shingles

ETIOLOGY AND PATHOGENESIS

Primary infection with varicella zoster virus (VZV) produces chickenpox in childhood, while reactivation of latent VZV in later life produces herpes zoster (shingles). VZV is highly contagious and transmission is believed to be predominantly through the inspiration of contaminated droplets. During the 2-week incubation period of primary infection, the virus proliferates within macrophages, with subsequent viremia and dissemination to the skin and other organs. VZV progress along the sensory nerves to the nerve ganglia, where it resides in a latent form.

Reactivation of latent VZV characteristically follows immunosuppression due to malignancy, drug administration, or HIV infection. Radiation or surgery of the spinal cord may also trigger secondary infection.

CLINICAL FEATURES

Chickenpox is characterized by the appearance of a maculopapular skin rash. Typically lesions arise on the trunk and spread to the face and limbs. The skin lesions may be preceded or accompanied by small (less than 5 mm diameter) oral ulcers in the palate and fauces.

The reactivation of VZV in herpes zoster produces severe pain that is followed within 24 hours by the appearance of vesiculobullous lesions (**85–87**). The trigeminal nerve is affected in about 15% of cases of zoster. The vesicular eruption is characteristically unilateral and limited to the mucosa and skin of one division of the trigeminal nerve. The infection heals with scarring but some patients may develop post-inflammatory pigmentation and residual sensory deficit.

DIAGNOSIS

The clinical presentation is usually sufficiently characteristic to enable diagnosis. Confirmation of infection can be made by virus isolation in cell culture or immunofluorescence on a smear from a recent lesion.

MANAGEMENT

Chickenpox does not usually require any treatment, although bed rest and patient isolation are advised during the active phase of the disease.

Although shingles is self-limiting, antiviral therapy should be considered in cases that present within the first 48 hours of onset of symptoms. Treatment with acyclovir (aciclovir) (800 mg tablet, 5 times daily for 7–10 days) has been the treatment of choice. However, the use of either

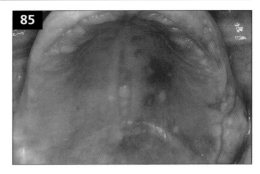

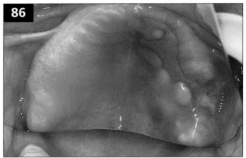

85, 86 Unilateral lesions of recurrent varicella zoster virus infection.

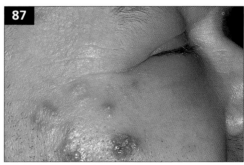

87 Vesicular eruption of herpes zoster on the skin.

valacyclovir (valaciclovir) (1 g 3 times daily) or famciclovir (500 mg 3 times daily) is now being employed in some countries. Therapy should be instituted as early as possible in the disease course, preferably before the development of vesicles. Approximately 15% of patients with shingles experience post-herpetic neuralgia and it is thought that provision of an antiviral therapy may reduce the likelihood of this complication.

Hand, foot, and mouth disease

ETIOLOGY AND PATHOGENESIS

The Coxsackie viruses are subdivided into Group A and Group B. Several Coxsackie viruses can produce painful orofacial conditions. Hand, foot, and mouth disease is usually caused by Coxsackie virus type A16 but may also be due to infection with types A4, A5, A9, and A10.

CLINICAL FEATURES

As the name of the condition implies, the characteristic distribution of lesions involves macular and vesicular eruptions on the hands (**88**), feet (**89**), and mucosa of the pharynx, soft palate, buccal sulcus, and tongue (**90**). Signs and symptoms are usually asymptomatic and resolve within 7–10 days.

DIAGNOSIS

Diagnosis is based on the clinical findings and history. It is important to differentiate this condition from primary herpes gingivostomatitis or varicella zoster infection. The relatively mild symptoms, cutaneous distribution, and epidemic spread help separate this condition from other conditions. Virus culture or detection of circulating antibodies may be employed to confirm clinical diagnosis.

MANAGEMENT

The self-limiting nature of the disease and the lack of virus-specific therapy limits treatment of hand, foot, and mouth disease to symptomatic measures. A bland mouthwash, such as sodium bicarbonate in warm water or chlorhexidine, alleviates oral discomfort. Analgesics may also be necessary for pain relief.

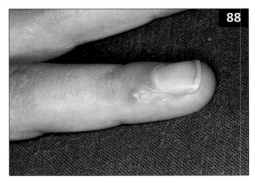

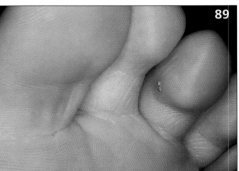

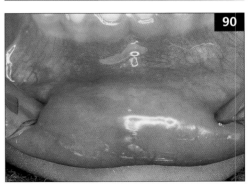

88–90 Vesicular eruptions of hand, foot, and mouth disease.

Herpangina

ETIOLOGY AND PATHOGENESIS
Herpangina is caused by infection with Coxsackie virus type A1, A2, A3, A4, A5, A6, A8, A10, A16, A22, or B3. The condition is usually spread by contaminated saliva. Infection is usually endemic, with outbreaks occurring in summer or early autumn. It occurs more often in children than in adults.

CLINICAL FEATURES
Patients complain of malaise, fever, dysphagia, and sore throat. A vesicular eruption appears on the soft palate, fauces, and tonsils (**91**). A diffuse erythematous pharyngitis is also a frequent feature. The clinical outcome is variable but resolution can be expected within 7–10 days, even in the absence of treatment.

DIAGNOSIS
Clinical appearance is usually diagnostic. Culture for Coxsackie viruses is not widely available and therefore diagnosis is based on demonstration of increased convalescent antibody levels.

MANAGEMENT
Treatment involves bed rest and the use of an antiseptic mouthwash. Patients should be encouraged to maintain adequate fluid intake.

Epidermolysis bullosa

ETIOLOGY AND PATHOGENESIS
Epidermolysis bullosa encompasses a group of uncommon bullous conditions which are inherited in either an autosomal dominant or a recessive pattern.

CLINICAL FEATURES
All forms of the disease are characterized by fragility of the epithelium of the mouth or skin accompanied by bulla formation (**92**). The severity of disease ranges from minor problems in the 'simple' and 'dystrophic' forms to severe involvement and possible death in the 'lethalis' form. Oral and perioral scar tissue can limit movement of the lips, tongue, and mouth.

DIAGNOSIS
Histopathologic examination demonstrates features of sub-epithelial bullae. In one form of the disease there is true lysis of basal cells and electron microscopy can aid diagnosis.

MANAGEMENT
Systemic steroid therapy has been found to limit bulla formation. Phenytoin therapy has been of some value, probably via an effect on fibroblast proliferation. Intra-oral lesions may develop after minor trauma and therefore great care should be taken during any dental treatment.

Mucocele

ETIOLOGY AND PATHOGENESIS
Mucocele is a clinical term that encompasses both a mucus extravasation phenomenon and a mucus retention cyst. Mucus extravasation results from the traumatic severing of a salivary gland duct to produce accumulation of saliva in the surrounding connective tissue, inflammation, and a granulation tissue wall. A mucus retention cyst results from obstruction of the salivary flow from a sialolith, periductal scar, or tumor. In contrast to mucus extravasation, the mucus in a retention cyst is contained within ductal epithelium.

CLINICAL FEATURES
Mucocele occurs most frequently on the lips. Other intra-oral sites that contain minor salivary glands and are prone to trauma may also be affected, such as the buccal mucosa and tongue. Clinically a mucocele presents as a painless, fluid-filled swelling with a blue discoloration and smooth surface (**93–95**). The size of swelling may range from a few millimeters to several centimeters. Mucus retention cysts develop less frequently than the mucus extravasation phenomenon.

DIAGNOSIS

Diagnosis of mucocele is established on history and examination. Ultimately, almost all lesions require surgical excision and this will enable diagnosis. In addition, differentiation between mucous retention and extravasation can only be made histopathologically.

MANAGEMENT

The treatment of both types of mucocele is surgical excision. Mucus aspiration has no last-ing benefit since the mucocele will quickly refill. Removal of the associated minor salivary glands forms an important part of the treatment in order to prevent recurrence. The placement of a silk suture in the roof of a large mucus retention cyst, particularly those arising in the floor of the mouth, can be useful to reduce its size prior to surgical excision.

Cryotherapy can be employed in children but there is a risk of recurrence.

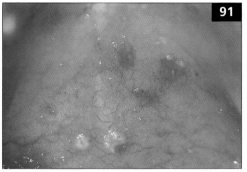

91 Blisters of herpangina in the palate.

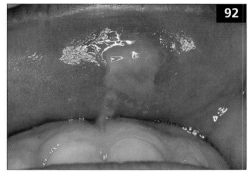

92 Blister of epidermolysis bullosa on upper labial mucosa.

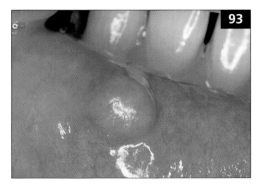

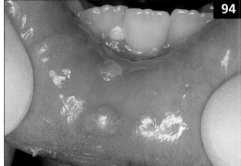

93–95 Mucocele.

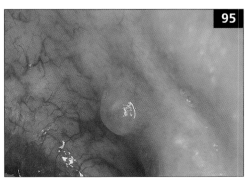

Erythema multiforme

ETIOLOGY AND PATHOGENESIS

This acute inflammatory condition is characterized by a variety of cutaneous lesions including bullae, papules, and macules. The cause of erythema multiforme is uncertain but has been associated with certain predisposing factors, including previous infection with herpes simplex virus or *Mycoplasma pneumoniae*, administration of certain systemic drugs, in particular sulfonamides and barbiturates, pregnancy, inflammatory bowel disease, and exposure to sunlight.

CLINICAL FEATURES

The orofacial lesions of erythema multiforme consist of blood-crusted lips (**96, 97**) and widespread painful oral ulceration (**98–101**). Skin involvement classically presents as concentric rings of erythema, the so-called 'target lesions' (**102–104**). The oral, ocular, and genital mucosa may be affected, either alone or in combination with the skin. The patient often has lymphadenopathy and feels generally unwell. The term 'Stevens–Johnson syndrome' has been used to describe severe cases with multiple sites of involvement including the skin, genital region, and the conjunctiva. The symptoms of erythema multiforme usually resolve spontaneously within 10–14 days. However, patients often experience two or three recurrences of reduced severity within 2–3 years of the initial episode.

DIAGNOSIS

Diagnosis of erythema multiforme is usually made easily due to the typical nature of the clinical presentation, especially when target lesions are present. The presence of crusting on the vermillion border of the lips is a particularly useful clinical sign. Primary herpetic gingivostomatitis is an important differential diagnosis to consider when involvement is limited to the oral mucosa.

MANAGEMENT

There is no specific treatment for erythema multiforme. If there is an association with recent drug therapy then this should be stopped. The provision of antiseptic mouthwash and, in severe cases, a short course of systemic steroid therapy has been found to be helpful. Oral prednisolone (prednisone) should be administered at a dose in the region of 40 mg daily for 3–4 days, gradually reduced over the following 7–10 days. Hospitalization may be necessary to ensure adequate hydration. It is important to obtain an ophthalmic opinion for patients with eye involvement because blindness is a potential problem. Patients with recurrent disease should undergo patch testing to exclude hypersensitivity to foodstuffs, particularly the benzoate-based preservatives (E210–E219). Long-term administration of aciclovir (acyclovir) (200 mg twice daily) has been found to prevent recurrent erythema multiforme in patients where herpes activity is thought to be a predisposing factor.

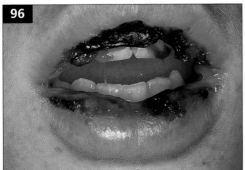

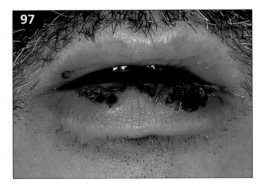

96, 97 Blood-crusted lips.

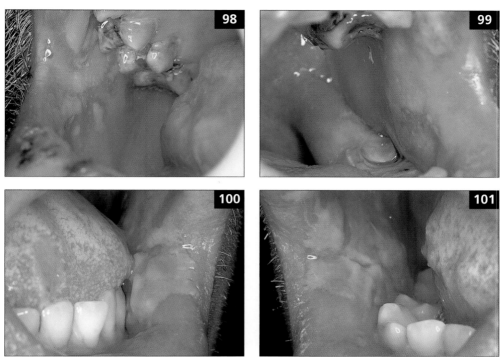

98–101 Widespread mucosal erosions of erythema multiforme.

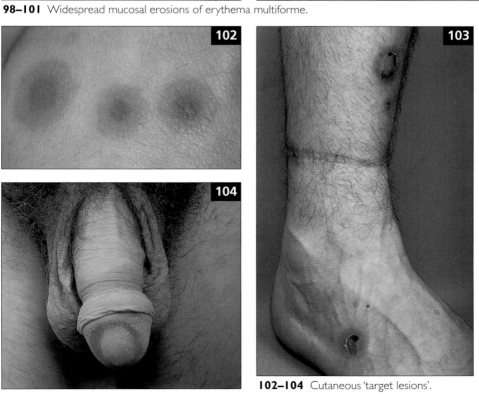

102–104 Cutaneous 'target lesions'.

Mucous membrane pemphigoid

ETIOLOGY AND PATHOGENESIS

Mucous membrane pemphigoid (MMP), an auto-immune vesiculobullous disease, can affect the oral mucosa. Immunoglobulins and components of complement are deposited along the basement zone producing the destruction of hemidesmosomes and the separation of the epithelium from the connective tissues. The antigenic targets are believed to be laminin 5 and a 180 kDa bullous pemphigoid antigen.

CLINICAL FEATURES

MMP is characterized by subepithelial bulla formation. Essentially there are two forms of pemphigoid and these are distinguished clinically by the site of involvement. In bullous pemphigoid, mucosal involvement is rare and cutaneous lesions predominate, whereas in MMP cutaneous involvement is rare. The oral presentation is variable but is often seen as areas of painful mucosal ulceration or desquamative gingivitis (**105–108**). Vesicles and bullae, which may be blood-filled, are rarely seen in the mouth due to early rupture (**109**). The patient is likely to describe their problem as 'the lining of the mouth peeling off'.

DIAGNOSIS

Biopsy tissue, sent for histopathologic analysis, should be examined for evidence of a submucosal split (**110**). Separate biopsy material should be sent on ice or in Michel's medium for direct immunofluorescence (IF) studies that will show a linear deposition of IgG and C_3 along the basement membrane (**111**). Indirect IF, using the patient's serum, is often negative and therefore of questionable additional value if direct IF is performed. Attempts to demonstrate Nikolsky's sign (mucosa lifting from the underlying connective tissue on pressure) should be resisted due to the production of further lesions.

MANAGEMENT

Steroid therapy forms the basis of treatment of pemphigoid, although there is a wide individual response to systemic or topical delivery. The majority of patients with MMP will respond to an initial course of systemic prednisolone (prednisone), followed by topical maintenance therapy. However, in some cases it may be necessary to maintain systemic oral steroids with the addition of azathioprine. Dapsone has also

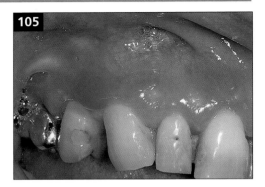

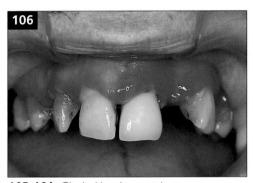

105, 106 Gingival involvement in mucous membrane pemphigoid.

been found to be effective in cases of MMP which do not respond to steroids. In addition, topical ciclosporin (cyclosporin) mouthwash or tacrolimus paste may be helpful.

An ophthalmic opinion is required as the condition is associated with the development of conjunctival scarring (**112**).

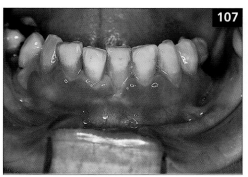
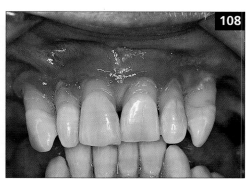

107, 108 Mucous membrane pemphigoid producing lesions of the full width of the attached gingivae.

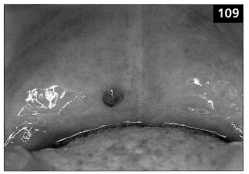
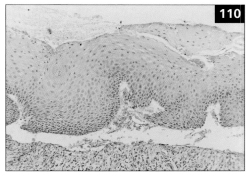

109 Blood-filled vesicle characteristic of mucous membrane pemphigoid.

110 H & E stain of a biopsy of oral mucosa showing a sub-epithelial split.

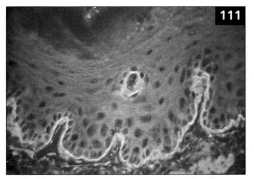
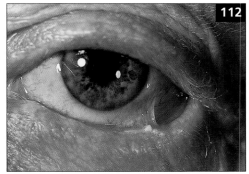

111 Direct immunofluorescence showing linear deposition of IgG along the basement membrane.

112 Symblepheron due to scar formation in the conjunctivae of a patient with mucous membrane pemphigoid. Both eyes were similarly affected.

Pemphigus

ETIOLOGY AND PATHOGENESIS

Pemphigus comprises a group of auto-immune, vesiculobullous disorders characterized by involvement of the skin, mouth, and other mucous membrane sites. Forms of pemphigus may be differentiated on the basis of the level of intra-epithelial involvement. Pemphigus vulgaris and pemphigus vegetans, the two forms that may produce oral lesions, affect the full width of the epithelium, while pemphigus foliaceous and pemphigus erythematosus occur in the upper prickle cell layer/spinous layer. Pemphigus arises because the patient develops circulating immunoglobulins directed towards the desmosomal region of the skin and mucous membranes. The antibody binding at these sites activates the complement and plasminogen activator leading to acantholysis, Tzanck cell formation, and development of vesicles.

CLINICAL FEATURES

The oral manifestations of pemphigus are nonspecific, with areas of erosion at any mucosal site (**113–115**). Nonkeratinized sites appear to be affected most often and vesicles are rarely seen due to early rupture (**116**). Skin lesions may or may not be present. Pemphigus vulgaris is usually a disease of older people, with females being more affected than males. The oral mucosa is involved initially in about 50% of cases of pemphigus vulgaris, and indeed oral involvement can precede involvement at other sites. Most cases are pemphigus vulgaris since pemphigus vegetans is extremely rare.

DIAGNOSIS

Attempts to demonstrate Nikolsky's sign (mucosa lifting from the underlying connective tissue on pressure) should be resisted due to the production of further lesions. Diagnosis is best confirmed by biopsy of an intact or recently ruptured bulla. Formalin fixed tissue should be sent for routine histopathology and fresh tissue should be sent for direct immunofluorescence. Routine pathology will show an intra-epithelial split (**117**). Direct immunofluorescence will show intercellular deposition of IgG (**118**). A blood sample should be sent for indirect immunofluorescence which may reveal the presence of circulating auto-antibody. The titer of circulating antibody is important since it reflects the degree of disease activity and can be used to monitor the effectiveness of therapy.

MANAGEMENT

Because the condition is a life-threatening disease, it is important to confirm clinical suspicion of its existence. If diagnosed, it is best to arrange immediate hospital admission to allow drug therapy to be commenced and monitored. Pemphigus vulgaris can rapidly involve large areas of skin and it is the protein loss and electrolyte disturbance associated with this aspect of the disease that is responsible for mortality. The drug therapy of choice is systemic prednisolone (prednisone) given at initial doses of up to 200 mg daily. Blood pressure needs careful monitoring in these early stages and antihypertensive drugs may be required. Once control is achieved then the dose of systemic steroid can be reduced to a maintenance level. Adjunctive azathioprine and cyclophosphamide have an important role in management since these drugs allow the dose of steroid to be reduced. Because pemphigus is a lifelong disease, therapy cannot be discontinued. Occasionally complications of long-term steroid therapy, such as cataracts and duodenal ulcers, can develop, and these need appropriate investigation and treatment.

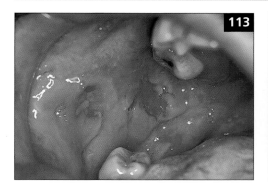

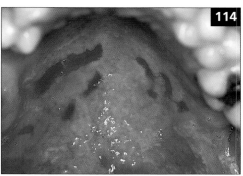

113–115 Extensive erosions of pemphigus vulgaris.

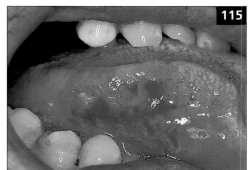

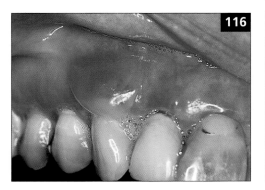

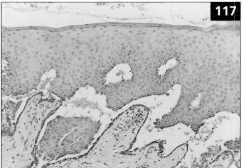

116 Bulla of pemphigus.

117 H & E stain of a biopsy of mucosa showing an intra-epithelial split.

118 Direct immunofluorescence showing inter-cellular deposition of IgG ('fish-net' appearance).

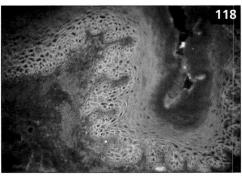

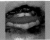

Linear IgA disease

ETIOLOGY AND PATHOGENESIS

The etiology of this condition is unknown. The condition shares many similarities with mucous membrane pemphigoid but it has also been proposed that linear IgA disease is a variant of dermatitis herpetiformis. However, unlike dermatitis herpetiformis, it is not associated with gluten-sensitive enteropathy and may not be responsive to dapsone therapy.

CLINICAL FEATURES

The disease produces persistent nonspecific oral ulceration and bullae are rarely present (**119**). Skin lesions also occur, particularly on the elbows, buttocks, and scalp.

DIAGNOSIS

Routine histopathologic investigations show nonspecific features and therefore the diagnosis is made by demonstration of a linear deposition of IgA along the basement membrane using direct immunofluorescence.

MANAGEMENT

Systemic steroid therapy produces clinical resolution of skin and oral lesions.

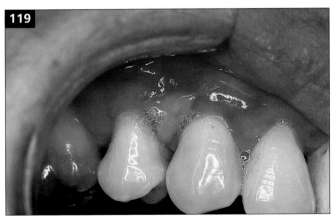

119 Erosion of the attached gingivae due to linear IgA disease.

Dermatitis herpetiformis

ETIOLOGY AND PATHOGENESIS
This condition has a relationship with celiac disease and involves hypersensitivity to the alpha gliadin fraction of wheat (gluten sensitivity).

CLINICAL FEATURES
Dermatitis herpetiformis is a rare chronic disease characterized by the development of crops of blisters on the skin or oral mucosa, which may be preceded by erythematous patches (**120, 121**). Lesions are exceedingly pruritic. As the name implies, there is a clinical similarity to herpetic lesions. Oral lesions are occasionally the first manifestation of the condition.

DIAGNOSIS
Histologic features are nonspecific but direct immunofluorescence will reveal a granular deposition of IgA along the basement membrane zone.

MANAGEMENT
Treatment is based on the use of dapsone or sulphapyridine (not available in the US). Elimination of gluten from the diet is an essential part of management.

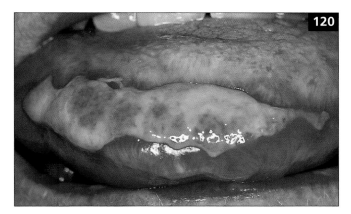

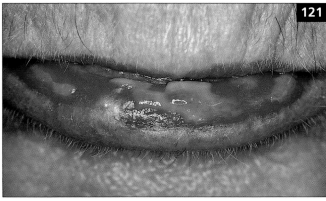

120, 121 Extensive erosions on the tip of the tongue and lower lip of a patient with dermatitis herpetiformis.

Angina bullosa hemorrhagica

ETIOLOGY AND PATHOGENESIS
The cause of angina bullosa hemorrhagica (ABH) is unknown, but it has been suggested that this blistering condition represents a mild and localized form of epidermolysis bullosa. In addition, an association between the use of steroid inhalers and ABH has been described. However, many patients presenting with ABH have no history of steroid therapy.

CLINICAL FEATURES
ABH is characterized by the rapid appearance of a solitary blood-filled blister (hemorrhagic bulla) usually in the soft palate (**122, 123**). Patients may complain of apparent tightness (angina) in the area immediately before and during the formation of swelling. The lesion invariably develops during eating and can be quite alarming to the patient, especially if hemorrhage

occurs. In these circumstances, the patient often seeks immediate medical or dental attention. However, by the time of presentation the bulla has usually spontaneously discharged to leave an area of erosion with blood at the periphery (**124, 125**).

DIAGNOSIS
Clinical history and appearance is often sufficient to make a diagnosis in an otherwise healthy patient. It is essential to exclude the presence of thrombocytopenia and therefore a full blood count to determine platelet levels should be undertaken.

MANAGEMENT
In the absence of any platelet deficiency the patient should be reassured and given an antiseptic mouthwash.

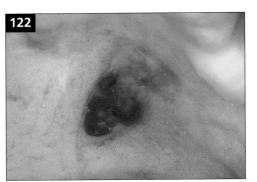

122 Angina bullosa hemorrhagica in the palate.

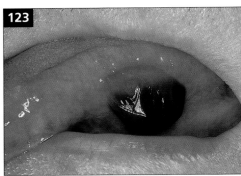

123 Angina bullosa hemorrhagica on the tongue.

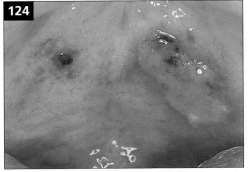

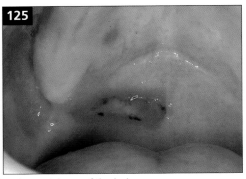

124, 125 Bullae of ABH rupture early to leave blood at the periphery of the lesion.

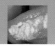

White Patches

- **General approach**
- **Lichen planus**
- **Lichenoid reaction**
- **Lupus erythematosus**
- **Chemical burn**
- **Pseudomembranous candidosis (thrush, candidiasis)**
- **Chronic hyperplastic candidosis (candidal leukoplakia)**
- **White sponge nevus**
- **Dyskeratosis congenita**
- **Frictional keratosis**
- **Nicotinic stomatitis (smoker's keratosis)**
- **Leukoplakia**
- **Squamous cell carcinoma**
- **Skin graft**
- **Hairy leukoplakia**
- **Pyostomatitis vegetans**
- **Submucous fibrosis**

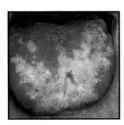
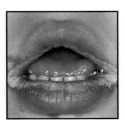
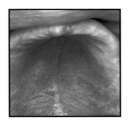
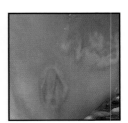

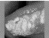

General approach

- White patches may develop within the oral mucosa due to trauma, infection, immune-related disease or neoplasia.
- White patches are usually painless, although discomfort can occur due to erosion or ulceration, particularly in lichen planus.
- Some white patches are pre-malignant and therefore biopsy should be routinely undertaken, unless there is no doubt of an alternative diagnosis.
- White patches may be localized or widespread throughout the mouth. Localized white patches suggest a traumatic or neoplastic etiology, while widespread involvement suggests a systemic, immunologic, or hereditary condition.

White patches may be divided into those that are painless and those that may be painful (*Table 3*).

Table 3 Patterns of white patches

White patches often associated with pain
- Lichen planus
- Lichenoid reaction
- Lupus erythematosus
- Chemical burn

White patches rarely associated with pain
- Pseudomembranous candidosis (candidiasis)
- Chronic hyperplastic candidosis (candidiasis)
- White sponge nevus
- Dyskeratosis congenita
- Frictional keratosis
- Nicotinic stomatitis
- Leukoplakia
- Squamous cell carcinoma
- Skin graft
- Hairy leukoplakia
- Pyostomatitis vegetans
- Submucous fibrosis

Lichen planus

ETIOLOGY AND PATHOGENESIS
Lichen planus is one of the more prevalent mucocutaneous disorders. The cause of lichen planus is not known, although it is immunologically mediated and resembles, in many ways, a hypersensitivity reaction to an unknown antigen. T-lymphocyte-mediated destruction of basal keratinocytes and hyperkeratinization produces the characteristic clinical lesions.

CLINICAL FEATURES
Lichen planus presents as white patches or striae that may affect any oral site, typically with a symmetric and bilateral distribution. Clinical appearance is variable and at least six forms have been described: reticular (**126–129**); papular; plaque-like (**130**); atrophic (**131, 132**); erosive (**133, 134**); and (rare) bullous. However, clear division among the different types is often difficult and examination of the mucosa of an individual patient may reveal that more than one

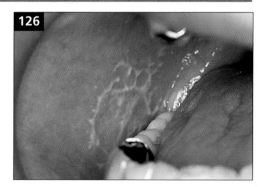

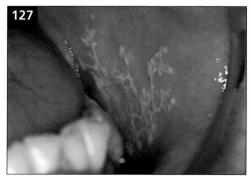

126, 127 Symmetrical reticular lichen planus in both buccal mucosae.

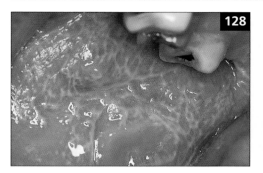

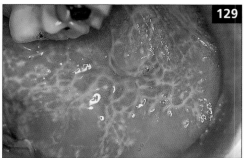

128, 129 Bilateral and symmetrical reticular lichen planus.

130 Plaque-like lichen planus on the dorsum of the tongue.

131 Atrophic lichen planus on the dorsum of the tongue.

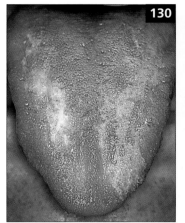

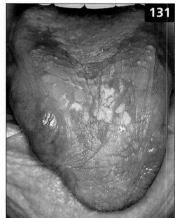

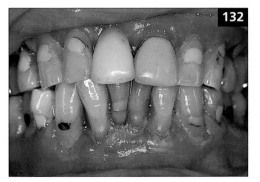

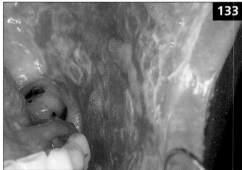

132 Atrophic lichen planus on the gingivae.

133 Erosive lichen planus on the buccal mucosa.

134 Erosive lichen planus on the gingivae.

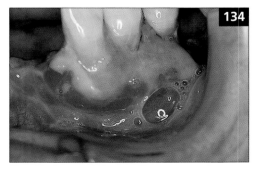

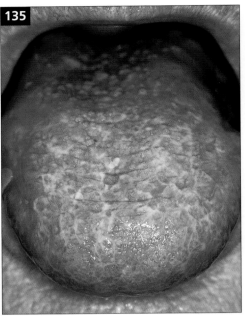

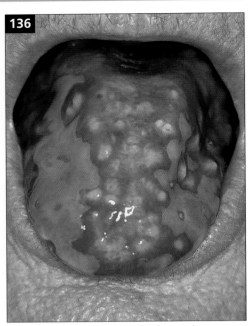

135–138 Chronologic change in the appearance of the tongue over a 4-year period in a patient with lichen planus.

subtype is present. In addition, the clinical signs and symptoms may change over a period of time (**135–138**).

The cutaneous lesions of lichen planus present as purple, pruritic papules that may develop at any site but most frequently occur on the flexor surfaces of the arms and legs (**139**). Fine white lines, known as Wickham's striae, may be seen on the surface of these papules. In contrast to the oral lesions which may be present for many years, skin involvement usually resolves within 18 months.

DIAGNOSIS

Clinical diagnosis of oral lichen planus is aided by the presence of cutaneous lesions. A mucosal biopsy will show a hyperkeratinized epithelium, basal cell destruction, and a dense band-like infiltrate of T-lymphocytes in the superficial connective tissue.

MANAGEMENT

The patient should be reassured of the benign nature of lichen planus. However, pre-existing lichen planus has occasionally been associated with the development of oral cancer, particularly if known risk factors are present. It is advisable to maintain regular reviews of such patients and

a biopsy should be performed if there is a change in clinical appearance.

The first line of treatment in symptomatic cases should consist of an antiseptic mouthwash combined with topical steroid therapy in the form of either hydrocortisone hemisuccinate pellets (2.5 mg) or betamethasone sodium phosphate (0.5 mg) allowed to dissolve on the affected area 2–4 times daily. Other preparations of topical steroid therapy, such as sprays, mouthwashes, creams, and ointments have been found to be beneficial for some patients. Intra-lesional injections of triamcinolone have also been tried with variable success. A short course of systemic steroid therapy may be required to alleviate acute symptoms in cases involving widespread ulceration, erythema, and pain. Other drugs used in lichen planus include ciclosporin (cyclosporin) mouthwash, topical tacrolimus, and systemic mycophenolate.

The possibility of coexisting oral candidosis (candidiasis) should be investigated and, if present, appropriate systemic antifungal agents prescribed. Furthermore, stress may be a precipitating factor, especially in older patients, and therefore anxiolytic therapy such as a tricyclic antidepressant may be helpful in selected situations.

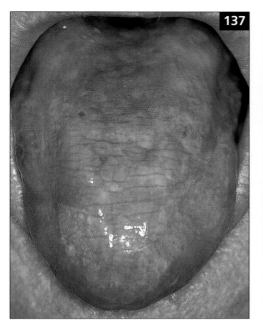

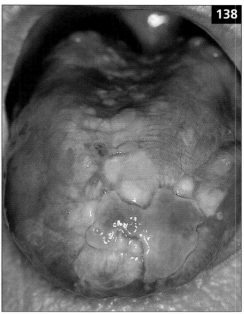

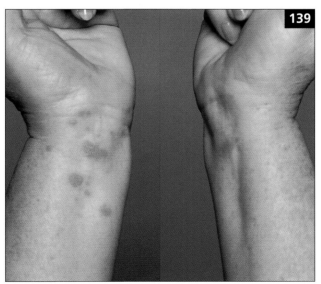

139 Cutaneous lesions of lichen planus on the flexor surface of the wrists.

Lichenoid reaction

ETIOLOGY AND PATHOGENESIS

Lichenoid reactions are so named because of the similarity, both clinically and histologically, to lichen planus. Systemic drugs, especially anti-hypertensives, hypoglycemics, and non-steroid anti-inflammatory agents, have been implicated in lichenoid reactions. In addition, direct contact with dental restorative materials has been shown to produce localized lichenoid lesions.

CLINICAL FEATURES

Lesions can occur at any intra-oral site, but in contrast to lichen planus it has been suggested that the distribution tends to be asymmetrical and may involve the palate, a site not associated with lichen planus (**140, 141**).

DIAGNOSIS

If oral lesions develop within a few weeks of the institution of drug therapy then there is likely to be a connection. Alternatively, if the distribution of lesions matches the position of old amalgams, a hypersensitivity to amalgam should be considered (**142**). More recently lichenoid reactions to composite materials have been reported. Mucosal biopsy is often helpful in supporting the diagnosis of a lichenoid reaction, although the changes may be difficult to differentiate from lichen planus or may be nonspecific. It has been suggested that indirect immunofluorescence may be of help in diagnosing a drug-induced lichenoid reaction, but this type of investigation is rarely employed.

MANAGEMENT

If the patient is taking a medicine known to be associated with the occurrence of lichenoid lesions, consideration should be given to a change of therapy to a structurally unrelated drug with similar therapeutic effect. In the absence of obvious precipitating factors then cutaneous patch testing may be helpful in identifying potential allergens, which then can be excluded. In the case of a reaction to amalgam, patch testing often detects a hypersensitivity to mercury and ammoniated mercury. Replacement of the amalgam restorations with alternative materials will result in the resolution of mucosal lesions within a few weeks. In the short term, topical anti-inflammatory agents or steroids can relieve symptoms.

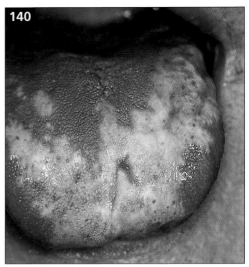

140 Lichenoid drug reaction with asymmetric distribution on the tongue.

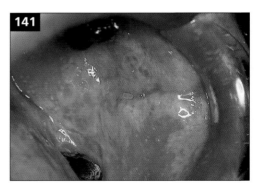

141 Lichenoid drug reaction with asymmetric distribution on the buccal mucosa.

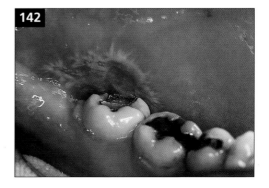

142 Lichenoid drug reaction on the buccal mucosa related to hypersensitivity to amalgam.

Lupus erythematosus

ETIOLOGY AND PATHOGENESIS

Lupus erythematosus is a chronic auto-immune disorder characterized by the production of anti-nuclear auto-antibodies. Immune complexes are formed and deposited along the basement membrane, leading to basal cell damage. In systemic lupus erythematosus (SLE) there is multi-system organ involvement resulting in kidney, pulmonary, cardiac, and joint disease. In discoid lupus erythematosus (DLE) the disease is confined to the skin but oral lesions develop in 15% of sufferers.

CLINICAL FEATURES

Patients with DLE have discrete, raised, erythematous, scaly patches and plaques on sun-exposed skin that progress to atrophic hypopigmented scars. The oral lesions of lupus erythematosus consist of localized striated, keratotic, and erythematous patches that resemble lichen planus (**143**). The most striking sign of SLE is a butterfly rash on the skin of the malar processes. Many patients with SLE also suffer from xerostomia and xerophthalmia and fulfil the criteria for secondary Sjögren's syndrome.

DIAGNOSIS

Serologic evidence of auto-antibodies is important for the diagnosis of SLE. Histologic examination of the oral mucosa shows basal cell destruction, basement membrane thickening, and lymphocytic infiltrates in the superficial connective tissues and in a perivascular distribution. Immunofluorescence shows granular immune deposits along the basement membrane (lupus band test).

MANAGEMENT

Symptomatic intra-oral DLE can be managed in a similar manner to oral lichen planus. Specifically, the first line of treatment should consist of an antiseptic mouthwash combined with topical steroid therapy in the form of either hydrocortisone hemisuccinate pellets (2.5 mg) or betamethasone sodium phosphate (0.5 mg) allowed to dissolve on the affected area 2–4 times daily. Other formats of topical steroid therapy such as sprays, mouthwashes, creams, and ointments have been found to be beneficial for some patients. Intra-lesional injections of triamcinolone have also been tried, with variable success. The antimalarial drugs, hydroxychloroquine and dapsone, have also been used successfully to managed oral DLE. In severe cases, characterized by widespread ulceration, erythema and pain, a short course of systemic steroid therapy may be required to alleviate acute symptoms.

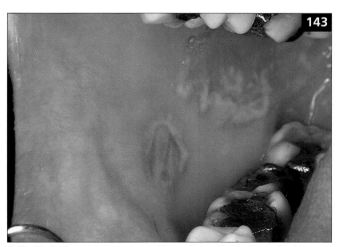

143 Radiating white patches with erythema in the buccal sulcus, which is characteristic of the oral lesions of lupus erythematosus.

Chemical burn

ETIOLOGY AND PATHOGENESIS
A superficial chemical injury of the oral mucosa will develop due to topical application of aspirin. Some patients attempt to treat an area of oral discomfort or toothache by the application of aspirin directly to the affected site. Patients may also place preparations based on aspirin on the fitting surface of dentures in order to relieve discomfort. The low pH of aspirin causes erythema and tissue necrosis and, with increasing contact time, coagulative necrosis. Eventually there is the formation of a white slough on the surface.

CLINICAL FEATURES
Chemical burns appear as a white, friable slough that can be easily removed, leaving a bed of erythema and ulceration. The most frequently involved site is the buccal sulcus or alveolar attached gingivae (**144**). Alternatively, chemical burns may be seen under a full denture.

DIAGNOSIS
Diagnosis is established on clinical examination and a history of aspirin application. A biopsy is not usually required but if performed will show nonspecific ulceration and fibrinous exudate.

MANAGEMENT
For most patients healing will begin once the application of the chemical has ceased. It is important to keep the mouth clean using an antiseptic mouthwash or bicarbonate of soda rinse several times a day until healing occurs.

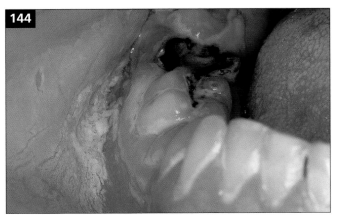

144 Aspirin burn seen as white slough adjacent to a grossly carious molar tooth. The patient had placed an aspirin tablet, at regular intervals, adjacent to the carious molar tooth in an attempt to relieve extreme pain.

Pseudomembranous candidosis (thrush, candidiasis)

ETIOLOGY AND PATHOGENESIS

Approximately 40% of the population harbor candida intra-orally in small numbers as members of the normal commensal oral microflora. Oral candidosis (candidiasis) has been described as 'the disease of the diseased' because proliferation of candida within the mouth is usually due to the presence of an underlying illness. The spectrum of candidal species which can exist in the oral cavity includes *Candida albicans, C. glabrata, C. tropicalis, C. pseudotropicalis, C. guillerimondi, C. dubliniensis,* and *C. krusei.* The majority of cases of thrush are due to *C. albicans,* although the use of chromogenic culture media in recent years has revealed an increase in the isolation of non-albicans species.

Age is an important factor in the development of oral candidosis (candidiasis) since thrush affects approximately 5% of newborn infants and 10% of elderly debilitated individuals. Thrush occurring in adulthood is usually due to the presence of iron deficiency (sideropenia), a blood dyscrasia, HIV infection, or secondary to antibiotic or steroid drug therapy.

CLINICAL FEATURES

Pseudomembraneous candidosis (candidiasis) is characterized by soft creamy-yellow patches that affect large areas of the oral mucosa, in particular the junction of the hard and soft palate (**145, 146**). Involvement is often limited when associated with inhaler therapy (**147**). Such plaques can be wiped off to reveal an underlying erythematous mucosa.

DIAGNOSIS

A smear of suspected thrush should be taken and stained by Gram's stain or periodic acid-Schiff reagent to demonstrate large numbers of fungal hyphae or blastospores. A swab or oral rinse should be taken and sent for culture.

MANAGEMENT

Management of pseudomembranous candidosis (candidiasis) is based primarily on the identification and eradication of any predisposing factor. The use of topical polyene agents such as amphotericin, nystatin, and miconazole, which are available in a variety of formulations, is of limited benefit. The new generation of imidazole derivative antifungal agents, such as fluconazole and itraconazole, are extremely effective within 7–15 days, although clinical infection will return after discontinuation of therapy if the underlying factors are not eliminated.

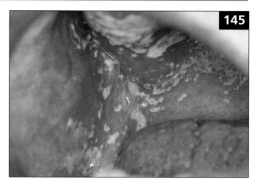

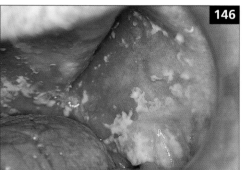

145, 146 Widespread pseudomembranous candidosis (candidiasis).

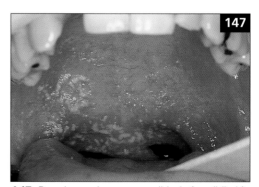

147 Pseudomembranous candidosis (candidiasis) in the soft palate related to steroid inhaler use.

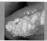

Chronic hyperplastic candidosis (candidal leukoplakia)

ETIOLOGY AND PATHOGENESIS

Risk factors for chronic hyperplastic candidosis (candidiasis) are similar to pseudomembraneous candidosis (candidiasis), although this form is particularly related to tobacco use. It is still uncertain if candidal invasion is the primary etiology or whether infection with candida is secondary to the formation of an altered epithelium. However, clinical resolution following the eradication of infection would support a primary role for candida. Occasionally, hyperplastic candidosis (candidiasis) includes elements of epithelial dysplasia and there is a recognized risk of malignant transformation.

CLINICAL FEATURES

Chronic hyperplastic candidosis (candidiasis) appears as thickened, irregular or smooth, white plaques, most frequently at the commissures of the mouth (**148**, **149**) or the dorsum of the tongue (**150**). In contrast to pseudomembraneous candidosis (candidiasis), the white plaques do not rub off. This form of candidosis (candidiasis) may occur in a mucocutaneous syndrome (**151**).

DIAGNOSIS

A mucosal biopsy of the affected mucosa should be performed. Histologic examination shows the presence of candidal hyphae within the keratin layers of hyperplastic epithelium accompanied by a chronic inflammatory cell infiltrate. An imprint culture should be taken from tissue immediately adjacent to the biopsy site. The imprint should not involve the actual area of mucosa to be removed since the surface layers will be disrupted and this may subsequently complicate the histopathologic interpretation of the biopsy material.

MANAGEMENT

In the past, prolonged topical polyene antifungal therapy for up to 3 months has been employed, with little benefit. More recently, however, the use of systemic antifungal agents has been found to produce clinical and histologic resolution in 2–3 weeks. Surgical excision may be necessary for persistent lesions with signs of epithelial dysplasia. The patient should be advised to stop any tobacco habit since lesions are likely to recur if smoking is not eliminated.

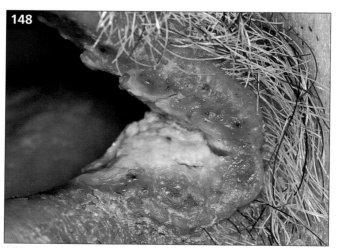

148 Chronic hyperplastic candidosis (candidiasis) presenting as an indurated ulcer with slough. The appearance raised some concern clinically that the lesion was a carcinoma.

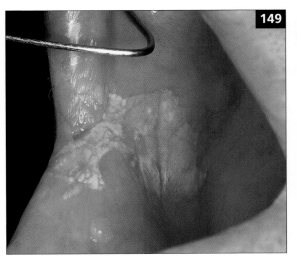

149 Chronic hyperplastic candidosis (candidiasis) in the commisure region.

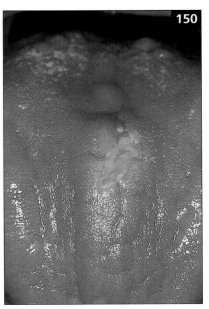

150 Chronic hyperplastic candidosis (candidiasis) presenting as a persistent white patch in the midline of the tongue.

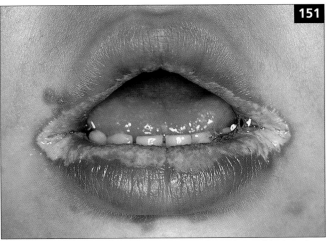

151 Persistent white patches on the lips of a patient with chronic mucocutaneous syndrome.

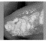

White sponge nevus

ETIOLOGY AND PATHOGENESIS

White sponge nevus is a benign condition that is inherited in an autosomal dominant fashion, although its expression is variable. It is due to point mutations of the keratin 4 and 13 genes.

CLINICAL FEATURES

The condition is asymptomatic and characterized by deeply-folded white lesions at several mucosal sites, particularly the buccal mucosa (**152–154**). Other sites in the body may be involved, including the mucosa of the vagina, vulva, anus, and esophagus, although developmental in origin, white sponge nevus is not usually first noticed until the second decade of life.

DIAGNOSIS

Diagnosis is made on the clinical presentation and history, especially the involvement of other family members. The biopsy shows hyperkeratosis with edematous keratinocytes showing peri-nuclear condensation of keratin. There is no epithelial dysplasia.

MANAGEMENT

No treatment is required since the condition is benign with no malignant potential. Occasional reports in the literature have suggested a symptomatic improvement following topical antibiotic therapy, but the basis and usefulness of this approach is uncertain.

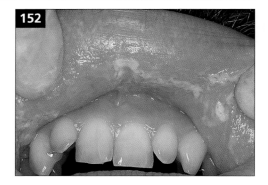

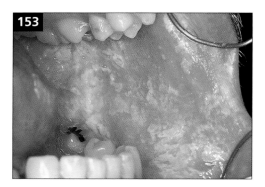

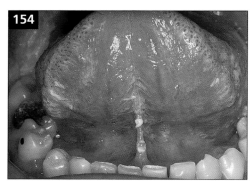

152–154 Widespread involvement of the oral mucosa in a patient with white sponge nevus.

Dyskeratosis congenita

ETIOLOGY AND PATHOGENESIS

Dyskeratosis congenita is an inherited syndrome in which patients undergo premature aging and have a predisposition to malignancy. X-linked and autosomal, both dominant and recessive, forms of the disease are recognized. The gene responsible for X-linked dyskeratosis congenita encodes a protein called dyskerin, which is abnormal. Afflicted individuals also show reduced telomere lengths of peripheral blood cells.

CLINICAL FEATURES

The clinical manifestations of dyskeratosis congenita become evident in the first 10 years of life. Reticulated skin hyperpigmentation of the upper chest and dysplastic nail changes characterize the cutaneous manifestations. Within the mouth, mucosal erosions and areas of leukoplakia, which are potentially malignant, may develop (155). Approximately 30% of the leukoplakia lesions progress to oral cancer in 10–30 years. Rapidly progressing periodontal disease, thrombocytopenia, and aplastic anemia may also be seen.

DIAGNOSIS

Diagnosis of dyskeratosis congenita is made on the history and clinical presentation. The biopsy of oral lesions is nonspecific, showing hyperkeratosis with epithelial atrophy and varying severity of dysplasia.

MANAGEMENT

The condition is managed symptomatically with careful observation of the oral mucosa and biopsy of suspicious areas to detect possible malignant transformation. The systemic manifestations are managed medically.

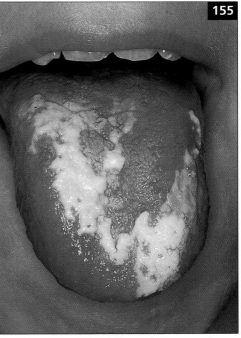

155 Dysplastic leukoplakia on the tongue of a patient with dyskeratosis congenita.

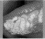

Frictional keratosis

ETIOLOGY AND PATHOGENESIS
Frictional keratosis develops due to chronic irritation of the oral mucosa. It is analogous to a callous which forms on an area of skin that is chronically rubbed. The most frequent cause of irritation in the mouth is the trauma of eating or chewing.

CLINICAL FEATURES
Any site in the mouth can be affected, the most common sites being the lips, lateral borders of the tongue, buccal mucosa at the occlusal line (**156, 157**) and an edentulous ridge (**158**). The lesion may be well-demarcated or diffuse, depending on the cause. The surface is homogeneously white but may have a thickened, corrugated appearance.

DIAGNOSIS
Diagnosis is based on the history and clinical appearance. A biopsy is often needed to confirm the diagnosis and rule out a neoplastic or inflammatory process. Microscopy shows hyperkeratosis without dysplasia and scattered chronic inflammatory cells in the underlying connective tissues.

MANAGEMENT
Treatment is directed at removing the cause of chronic irritation. Rough surfaces on the teeth or the components of any denture need to be corrected. Sometimes, the provision of an acrylic guard to be worn at night can help to prevent cheek and lip chewing. There is no evidence that chronic trauma alone predisposes to the development of malignancy.

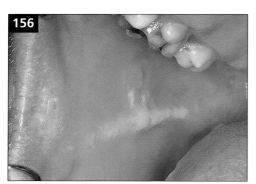

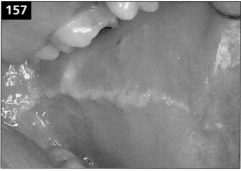

156, 157 Frictional keratosis presenting as bilateral linear white patches in the buccal mucosa at the occlusal line.

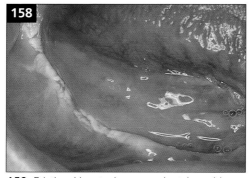

158 Frictional keratosis on an edentulous ridge.

Nicotinic stomatitis (smoker's keratosis)

ETIOLOGY AND PATHOGENESIS
Nicotinic stomatitis is the most frequently occurring tobacco-related keratosis in the mouth. It can be associated with pipe, cigar, or cigarette smoking. The severity of the condition is proportional to the amount of the tobacco product that is used. The hyperkeratosis of nicotinic stomatitis is reactive to the heat generated by the tobacco product and the chemicals present.

CLINICAL FEATURES
The characteristic site of involvement is the hard palate. Although predominantly white, there are areas of erythema with punctate red dots representing inflamed minor salivary duct orifices (**159**). If a denture is worn, this will protect the covered mucosa in the hard palate and produce an obvious distinction between affected and nonaffected areas (**160**).

DIAGNOSIS
Diagnosis is based on the history of tobacco product use and the clinical appearance. A biopsy is usually not indicated since the risk of neoplastic transformation is low.

MANAGEMENT
The patient should discontinue the tobacco habit. On the hard palate the condition is benign, although it is an important indicator of tobacco use and may indicate a risk of dysplasia and neoplasia at other susceptible sites, in particular the floor of the mouth, the lateral margin of the tongue, or the retro-molar region.

159 Nicotinic stomatitis in the palate.

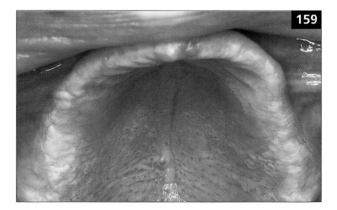

160 Nicotinic stomatitis in the posterior region of palate with a lack of involvement in the anterior tissues which are normally covered by an upper denture.

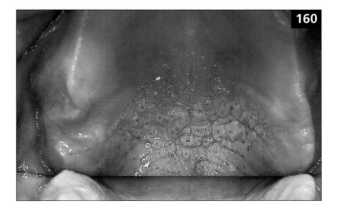

Leukoplakia

ETIOLOGY AND PATHOGENESIS

Leukoplakia is a clinical term used to describe 'a white patch or plaque on the oral mucosa that cannot be rubbed off and cannot be characterized clinically as any specific disease'. This definition therefore excludes conditions such as lichen planus, white sponge nevus, and pseudomembranous candidosis (candidiasis). Most cases of leukoplakia are associated with a tobacco habit, although alcohol, invasive candidal infection, hematinic deficiency (Plummer–Vinson syndrome), and chronic trauma may also play a role. In developed countries, the transformation rate of leukoplakia to oral cancer is low at 1–2% in 5 years, but this may increase to 15–20% in the Indian sub-continent.

CLINICAL FEATURES

Most cases of leukoplakia occur in the middle-aged and older populations. The most frequently affected sites are the tongue, lower lip, retromolar region, and floor of the mouth (161–164). Leukoplakia in the floor of the mouth has a higher rate of malignant transformation than other sites. Clinically, leukoplakia may have a range of appearances from flat white patches, wart-like lesions, and thickened leathery patches, to mixed red/white patches, so-called 'speckled leukoplakia' (165).

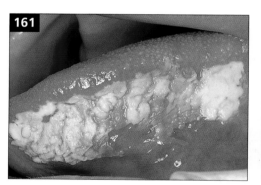

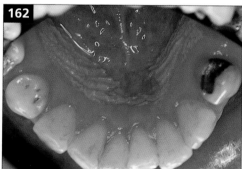

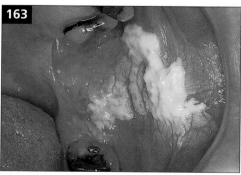

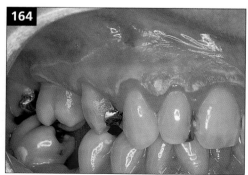

161–164 Various appearances of intra-oral leukoplakia.

DIAGNOSIS

A biopsy of a leukoplakia is mandatory since lesions with similar clinical appearance have a range of differing histologic diagnoses, including carcinoma. In addition, it essential to determine the severity of any epithelial dysplasia that may be present.

MANAGEMENT

In the absence of dysplasia, no treatment is required apart from periodic re-examination every 6 months to assess for any clinical change that would indicate a need to re-biopsy. The management of lesions with dysplastic changes will depend on the severity of the epithelial dysplasia. A mildly dysplastic leukoplakia may be managed conservatively with emphasis on the elimination of tobacco or alcohol habits, treatment of any candidal infection, and exclusion of any underlying hematinic deficiency. The provi-sion of long-term retinoid therapy has been suggested to have a role in the management of mild dysplasia. However, recent evidence shows that although retinoid therapy improves the clinical appearance of the lesions, genetic aberrations remain unaltered. Therefore, the efficacy of this therapy has been questioned. Re-biopsy should be performed after 3 months to assess the effect of measures aimed at the correction of etiologic factors. Long-term review at 6-monthly intervals is required. The role of brush biopsy in monitoring such lesions is under review and may be helpful in the future. Although opinions do differ, severely dysplastic lesions should be managed as carcinoma due to the risk of malignant change (166, 167). The role of photodynamic therapy in the management of localized severe dysplasia and small carcinoma is presently being evaluated.

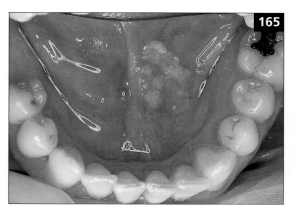

165 Speckled leukoplakia in the floor of the mouth.

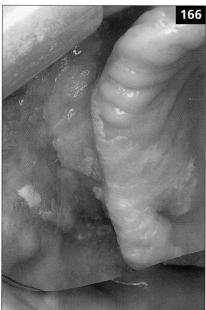

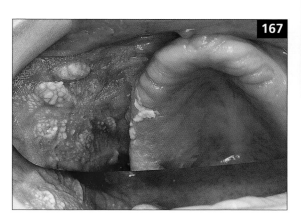

166, 167 Leukoplakia in the right buccal and palatal mucosa that underwent malignant change.

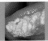

Squamous cell carcinoma

ETIOLOGY AND PATHOGENESIS
The use of tobacco and alcohol are the two most important risk factors for the development of oral squamous cell carcinoma (SCC) (Chapter 2, p. 28). Although it has been suggested that chewing tobacco is a significant cause of oral SCC, epidemiologic studies have shown that the risk is small and less than that associated with smoking tobacco. By contrast, the use of pan (areca nut and tobacco leaves soaked in lime) is significantly associated with the development of mucosal white patches and oral SCC. Prolonged and frequent exposure to the ultra-violet rays of the sun is the most important etiologic factor in SCC occurring on the lower lip.

CLINICAL FEATURES
SCC can occur at any intra-oral site, but the tongue, floor of the mouth, and retro-molar region are most frequently involved (**168, 169**). The hard palate is rarely involved. The vermillion border is the most frequent site for lip carcinoma, with the vast majority of cases occurring on the lower lip, reflecting its greater exposure to sunlight in comparison to the upper lip. SCC may present in a variety of mucosa changes including, as covered in this section, a white patch. SCC presenting as a white patch is usually painless and firm to palpation.

DIAGNOSIS
A biopsy should be undertaken of any white patch where there is uncertainty as to the cause. In most instances a biopsy of a suspicious lesion can be performed under local anesthesia. It is important that the biopsy is large enough and representative. Radiographs may be necessary to establish any change in the underlying bone.

MANAGEMENT
A patient diagnosed as having an oral SCC should be referred to a specialist cancer treatment center for assessment and treatment. Treatment will consist of either surgery or radiotherapy, or a combination of both forms of therapy (Chapter 2, p. 28).

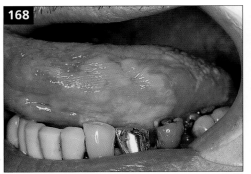
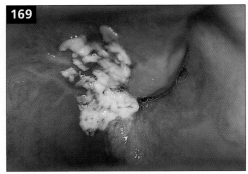

168, 169 Contrasting appearance of squamous cell carcinoma as a smooth white patch on the tongue compared to an exophytic lesion in the palate.

Skin graft

ETIOLOGY AND PATHOGENESIS

A section of skin from a donor site, usually the arm or thigh, is placed at a surgical site in the mouth to close a wound. Grafting is often used following excision of large areas of dysplasia or malignancy.

CLINICAL FEATURES

A skin graft appears as a white wrinkled area within the mouth. The transition from skin graft to mucosa is abruptly defined (**170**). If the graft is full-thickness and includes dermal appendages from the donor site, then hair may be present (**171, 172**).

DIAGNOSIS

Diagnosis is made on the history and clinical appearance. A thickening of the graft or change in colour may indicate the need for biopsy to rule out dysplasia or carcinoma.

MANAGEMENT

No treatment is required apart from observation, particularly if the patient has a previous history of oral cancer. Interestingly, it has recently been found that such skin grafts may become secondarily infected with candida. The significance of candidal infection is presently unknown.

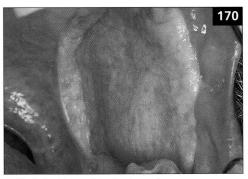

170 Split skin graft in the buccal mucosa.

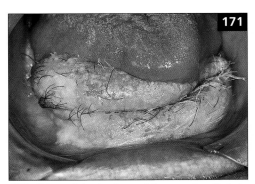

171 Skin graft in the floor of the mouth with hair.

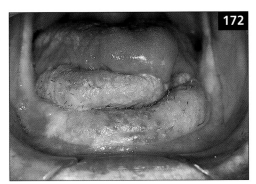

172 Skin graft in the floor of the mouth following 'haircut'.

Hairy leukoplakia

ETIOLOGY AND PATHOGENESIS

Hairy leukoplakia was first described in association with HIV infection and the frequency and severity of the lesions was related to the degree of immunosuppression. Subsequently, hairy leukoplakia has been described in patients with immunosuppression due to other reasons, in particular organ transplantation. Furthermore, a small number of cases of hairy leukoplakia has been reported in individuals with no apparent immunocompromised state. Hairy leukoplakia is considered an opportunistic infection caused by the Epstein–Barr virus (EBV) which infects keratinocytes within the mucosa. EBV particles can be found in the upper keratinocyte layers of all cases of hairy leukoplakia. It is not known why the lateral border of the tongue is the site of preferential involvement.

CLINICAL FEATURES

Hairy leukoplakia appears as a well-demarcated, corrugated white lesion varying from flat, plaque-like to papillary-villous (**173**). It occurs almost exclusively on the lateral border of the tongue and produces no symptoms (**174, 175**).

DIAGNOSIS

A biopsy is usually indicated when the diagnosis is not apparent clinically. The biopsy shows marked hyperparakeratosis with viral inclusions in the nuclei of superficial keratinocytes. Structures consistent with hyphae and spore forms of candida can often be seen in the keratin layers. *In situ* hybridization studies will reveal the presence of EBV in upper level keratinocytes.

MANAGEMENT

No treatment is usually needed for hairy leukoplakia since the condition is benign; it may produce a cosmetic problem only if it is large. Unsightly lesions can be treated with aciclovir (acyclovir), gancyclovir, tretinoin, or podophyllin, although the lesions invariably recur once therapy is discontinued. Improvement in the underlying immunosuppression frequently results in the regression of hairy leukoplakia.

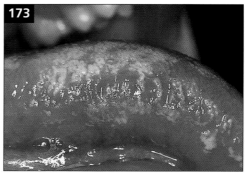

173 Classic presentation of hairy leukoplakia as a corrugated white patch on the lateral margin of the tongue.

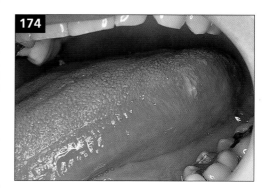

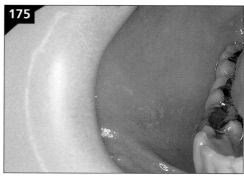

174, 175 Hairy leukoplakia on the lateral margin of the tongue and the buccal mucosa.

Pyostomatitis vegetans

ETIOLOGY AND PATHOGENESIS
Pyostomatitis vegetans is a chronic, pustular, mucocutaneous disorder most often seen in association with inflammatory bowel diseases, such as Crohn's disease and ulcerative colitis. The cause of the oral mucosal lesions is unknown.

CLINICAL FEATURES
This condition can occur anywhere in the mouth but is seen most frequently on the buccal or labial mucosa (176, 177). Erythema progresses to tiny yellow pustules measuring 2–3 mm in diameter and evolves to larger vegetating papillary lesions of friable mucosa. Males are affected twice as frequently as females and the condition is most often seen in the third to the sixth decades of life.

DIAGNOSIS
Diagnosis is made on clinical examination and the history of inflammatory bowel disease. Diagnosis is more difficult to achieve in the 25% of patients who have no bowel abnormalities. The biopsy of oral mucosa is nonspecific, showing chronically-inflamed mucosa, superficial abscesses, ulceration, and necrosis.

MANAGEMENT
If pyostomatitis vegetans occurs in association with inflammatory bowel disease, then successful management of the bowel involvement is accompanied by a marked improvement in the oral lesions. Indeed, remission of oral lesions reflects control of the bowel disorder. Oral lesions can also be treated with oral antiseptics, local corticosteroids, or systemic administration of the antimicrobial agent, metronidazole.

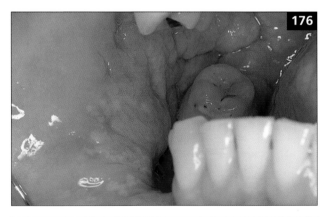

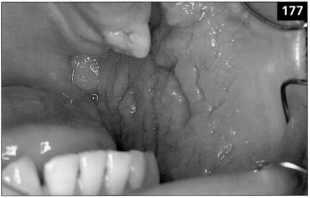

176, 177 Pyostomatitis vegetans producing erythema, yellow micro-abscesses, and fissuring within the buccal mucosa.

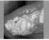

Submucous fibrosis

ETIOLOGY AND PATHOGENESIS
This condition is characterized by the development of fibrous tissue in the buccal mucosa and palate. The primary causative factor is chewing the areca (betel) nut. Although many patients with submucous fibrosis have a long history of areca nut use, the development of the condition does not appear to be dose-dependent. Other contributing factors include a chronic exposure to chilli peppers or prolonged deficiency of iron and vitamin B complexes, particularly folic acid. The primary abnormality in submucous fibrosis is a combination of excessive production and insufficient degradation of collagen by fibroblasts.

CLINICAL FEATURES
Submucous fibrosis mainly affects individuals from South-East Asia or India. It occurs in a wide age range but most suffers are 20–40 years old at the time of presentation. Irregular, flat, white lesions develop in the mouth, particularly the buccal mucosa (**178**), the soft palate, and also the esophagus and pharynx. The most striking feature is the formation of marked fibrous bands that can be palpated in the cheeks and the soft palate. These bands result in a loss of elasticity of the tissues and limited opening of the mouth (**179**).

DIAGNOSIS
Diagnosis is based on the manual detection of fibrous bands within the mouth and associated trismus. Biopsy often worsens the condition but may be necessary to determine if the white lesions contain epithelial dysplasia. It is important to differentiate this condition from fibrosis and scarring secondary to injury.

MANAGEMENT
A number of treatments have been proposed for the management of submucous fibrosis. The most important treatment is to have the patient discontinue all use of areca nut. For patients with restricted opening, manual stretching exercises can be helpful. Steroid injections directly into the fibrous bands of the buccal mucosae have been used. Similarly, enzymes that digest the fibrous tissues, such as chymotrypsin and hyaluronidase, have also been injected into the affected tissues. Finally, surgical procedures to excise and free the fibrous bands have also been tried, with mixed results. Since submucous fibrosis is associated with malignant change in the overlying epithelium, it is important that the patient is reviewed closely. Approximately one-third of patients with submucous fibrosis will develop oral cancer.

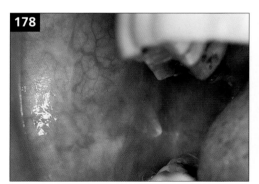

178 'Whitening' of the buccsal mucosa in association with submucous fibrosis.

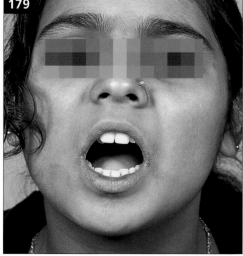

179 Restricted mouth opening due to fibrosis in the cheeks of a patient with submucous fibrosis.

Erythema

- **General approach**
- **Post-radiotherapy mucositis**
- **Contact hypersensitivity reaction**
- **Lichen planus**
- **Acute erythematous (atrophic) candidosis (candidiasis)**
- **Geographic tongue (benign migratory glossitis, erythema migrans)**
- **Median rhomboid glossitis (superficial midline glossitis)**
- **Angular cheilitis**
- **Iron deficiency anemia**
- **Pernicious anemia**
- **Folic acid (folate) deficiency**
- **Chronic erythematous (atrophic) candidosis (candidiasis)**
- **Erythroplakia**
- **Squamous cell carcinoma**
- **Infectious mononucleosis (glandular fever)**

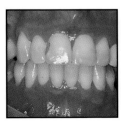
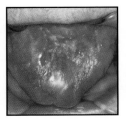
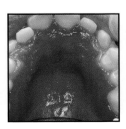
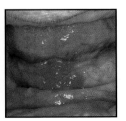

General approach

- Erythema of the oral mucosa may be due to trauma, infection, immune-related disease, or neoplasia.
- Most erythematous lesions within the mouth will cause a degree of discomfort, although this is not usually severe. Occasionally, erythematous lesions may be painless.
- Some erythematous patches are pre-malignant and therefore biopsy should be routinely undertaken unless there is no doubt about the diagnosis.
- Erythematous lesions affecting the oral mucosa are usually widespread.

Patterns of erythema are shown in *Table 4.*

Table 4 Patterns of erythema

Painful and may ulcerate
- Post-radiotherapy mucositis
- Contact hypersensitivity reaction
- Erosive lichen planus

Painful with no ulceration
- Acute erythematous candidosis (candidiasis)
- Geographic tongue
- Median rhomboid glossitis
- Angular cheilitis
- Iron deficiency anemia
- Pernicious anemia
- Folate deficiency

Painless with no ulceration
- Erythroplakia
- Chronic erythematous candidosis (candidiasis)

Painless and may ulcerate
- Squamous cell carcinoma
- Infectious mononucleosis

Post-radiotherapy mucositis

ETIOLOGY AND PATHOGENESIS
Ionizing radiation is used to treat many malignancies by targeting dividing cells. For oral squamous cell carcinoma, radiation is given in 2 Gy daily fractions up to about 70 Gy. The therapeutic effects of radiation are dose dependent, as are the complications. The effect of radiation is nonspecific and therefore normal cells undergoing division are also susceptible to the therapy. Basal epithelial cells, which divide frequently, are particularly susceptible to radiation, and this leads to a mucositis.

CLINICAL FEATURES
Typically, multiple painful red patches and areas of ulceration develop throughout the oral mucosa (**180, 181**). Nonkeratinized surfaces, such as the buccal mucosa and the floor of the mouth, are particularly susceptible to radiation damage. Mucositis usually begins 1–2 weeks after the start of radiation therapy. The condition persists for several weeks after the termination of treatment.

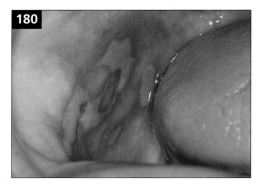

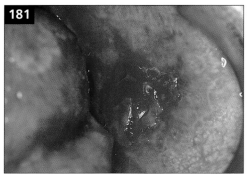

180, 181 Post-radiotherapy mucositis.

DIAGNOSIS

Diagnosis is made on clinical history and examination. Biopsy is not necessary and is generally contraindicated during the radiation treatment.

MANAGEMENT

Keeping the mouth clean is the most important aspect of management. Rinsing the mouth frequently with warm water and baking soda mouthwashes limits the likelihood of infection. Chlorhexidine mouthwash (0.2%) may also be used but a brown coloration often develops on the dorsum of the tongue. The chlorhexidine can be diluted in water up to 10-fold to reduce this problem and the discomfort experienced by some patients. Topical anesthetics may be necessary for painful lesions. Alcohol-containing mouthwashes are contraindicated since they cause further atrophy of the mucosa and pain. Investigations should be performed to determine the presence of any secondary candidosis (candidiasis) or staphylococcal infection. Appropriate antimicrobial therapy is required if culture detects infection.

Contact hypersensitivity reaction

ETIOLOGY AND PATHOGENESIS

A contact hypersensitivity reaction can be caused by an array of foreign materials, such as toothpastes, mouthwashes, candy, mint, chewinggum, cinnamon, topical antimicrobials, and essential oils. The condition is a cell-mediated immune response requiring antigen presentation by Langerhans cells to T-lymphocytes. It is important to note that a suspected reaction to the polymethylmethacrylate material of dentures is rarely a hypersensitivity phenomenon but is more often inflammation as a result of candidal infection.

CLINICAL FEATURES

Lesions due to contact allergy usually lie adjacent to the causative agent, particularly when associated with denture materials. Alternatively, reactions to foodstuffs, mouthwashes, or toothpastes may be diffuse (182). The lesions vary from erythematous patches that may show vesiculation to granular red patches.

DIAGNOSIS

History and examination are essential in making a diagnosis. This can be assisted by biopsy, although the histologic findings are often nonspecific. Cutaneous patch testing is helpful in diagnosis. Candidal infection can be excluded by the use of a swab or imprint culture of lesional mucosa.

MANAGEMENT

The primary treatment is to eliminate the cause of the allergic reaction which is usually followed by resolution within a few weeks. Topical corticosteroid treatment can help to reduce the presenting symptoms until the causative factor is corrected. Amalgam restorations can be replaced with composite materials or, in the case of a reaction to methylmethacrylate, a denture can be constructed using a nylon base.

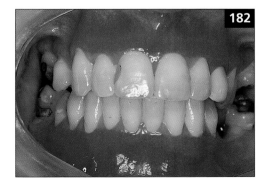

182 Erythema of the gingivae due to hypersensitivity to cinnamon in toothpaste.

Lichen planus

ETIOLOGY AND PATHOGENESIS

The cause of lichen planus is not known, although it is immunologically mediated and resembles, in many ways, a hypersensitivity reaction to an unknown antigen. T-lymphocyte-mediated destruction of the basal keratinocytes and hyperkeratinization produces the characteristic clinical lesions.

CLINICAL FEATURES

Lichen planus characteristically presents as white patches (Chapter 4, p. 60). However, the atrophic and erosive forms of the disease may produce erythematous lesions with or without white striae (**183–185**).

DIAGNOSIS

Diagnosis of this form of lichen planus is likely to require a biopsy.

MANAGEMENT

The first line of treatment in symptomatic cases should consist of an antiseptic mouthwash combined with topical steroid therapy in the form of either hydrocortisone hemisuccinate pellets (2.5 mg) or betamethasone sodium phosphate (0.5 mg) allowed to dissolve on the affected area 2–4 times daily. Other preparations of topical steroid therapy, such as sprays, mouthwashes, creams, and ointments, have been found to be beneficial for some patients. A short course of systemic steroid therapy may be required to alleviate acute symptoms in cases involving widespread ulceration, erythema, and pain. Other drugs used in lichen planus include ciclosporin (cyclosporin) mouthwash, topical tacrolimus, and systemic mycophenolate.

The possibility of coexisting oral candidosis (candidiasis) should be investigated and, if present, appropriate systemic antifungal agents prescribed. Stress may be a precipitating factor, especially in older patients, and therefore anxiolytic therapy, such as a tricyclic antidepressant, may be helpful in selected situations.

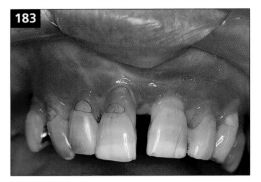

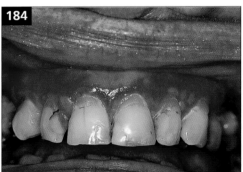

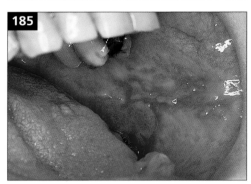

183–185 Erythema of the attached gingivae and buccal mucosa in erosive lichen planus.

Acute erythematous (atrophic) candidosis (candidiasis)

ETIOLOGY AND PATHOGENESIS

In the past the term atrophic has been used to describe this form of candidosis (candidiasis). However, it is now appreciated that the mucosa is not atrophic and therefore the term 'erythematous' is preferred. Factors that predispose to erythematous candidosis (candidiasis) include systemic antibiotic therapy, inhaled steroid therapy, and immunosuppression.

CLINICAL FEATURES

Acute erythematous candidosis (candidiasis) is characterized by the development of red areas of the oral mucosa. Although any intra-oral site may be affected, the midline of the palate (**186**) and the dorsum of the tongue (**187**) are most frequently involved. Unlike other forms of oral candidosis (candidiasis), acute erythematous candidosis (candidiasis) is often painful. This form of candidosis (candidiasis) may be an indication of underlying HIV infection.

DIAGNOSIS

A smear from the affected site may demonstrate the presence of candida. Alternatively, a swab or imprint culture should be taken and sent for culture.

MANAGEMENT

If the patient is taking antibiotic therapy, then consideration should be given to discontinuing this. Patients on steroid inhaler therapy should be advised to rinse or gargle with water after inhaler therapy to minimize the persistence of the drug in the oral cavity. The use of a systemic antifungal, such as fluconazole 50 mg daily for 7 days, should be considered if the patient is otherwise unwell or medically compromised. In the absence of any obvious cause, HIV infection should be suspected.

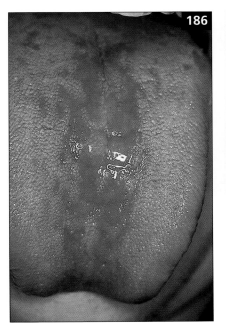

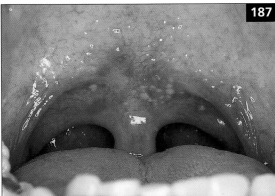

186, 187 Acute erythematous candidosis (candidiasis) at characteristic sites of dorsum of the tongue and the soft palate.

Geographic tongue (benign migratory glossitis, erythema migrans)

ETIOLOGY AND PATHOGENESIS

The etiology of geographic tongue is unknown. Although the mucosal condition resembles psoriasis histopathologically, no connection between the two entities has been proven. However, geographic tongue is seen approximately five times more frequently in patients with psoriasis compared to the normal population.

CLINICAL FEATURES

This condition is characterized by the appearance of irregular depapillated erythematous areas surrounded by pale well-demarcated margins on the dorsal surface and lateral margins of tongue (**188–190**). Such areas appear and regress relatively quickly over a period of a few days. Rarely, similar-appearing lesions can be found on other mucosal surfaces (**191**). The condition is relatively common and can affect any age, including young children. Patients are often unaware of the presence of geographic tongue, although some individuals complain of discomfort on eating, especially hot or spicy foods.

DIAGNOSIS

Geographic tongue can be diagnosed from the clinical appearance and history. Biopsy is rarely indicated but should be undertaken whenever the presence of a more sinister lesion is suspected.

MANAGEMENT

The patient should be reassured about the benign nature of the condition. Nutritional deficiency should be excluded in all patients with symptomatic geographic tongue. Therefore, a full blood count and an evaluation of levels of vitamin B_{12}, corrected whole blood folic acid (folate), and ferritin should be undertaken. In addition, a zinc assay may be helpful since symptomatic geographic tongue has been found to respond to topical zinc therapy. Zinc should be given as dispersible zinc sulfate (sulphate), 125 mg dissolved in water and used as a mouthwash for approximately 2–3 minutes every 8 hours over 3 months.

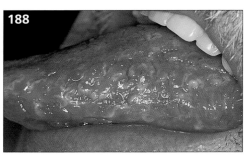

188–190 Variable appearance of geographic tongue.

191 Rare involvement of the buccal mucosa in a patient with geographic tongue.

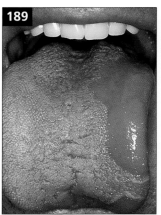

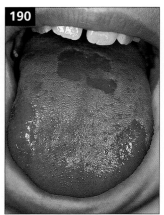

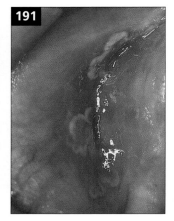

Median rhomboid glossitis (superficial midline glossitis)

ETIOLOGY AND PATHOGENESIS

Median rhomboid glossitis has long been considered to be a development abnormality associated with the persistence of the tuberculum impar. However, this theory has come into question since the condition is rare in children and presents mainly in adults. Moreover, recent evidence has shown that many of these lesions contain candida and clinical resolution occurs following systemic antifungal therapy.

CLINICAL FEATURES

Median rhomboid glossitis characteristically presents as a smooth well-demarcated area of erythema at the junction of the anterior two-thirds and posterior one-third of the tongue (**192, 193**). A similar erythematous patch, the so-called 'kissing lesion', can sometimes be seen on the adjacent hard palate.

DIAGNOSIS

Diagnosis can be made relatively easily from the clinical appearance. Microbiologic investigations should include an imprint culture from the tongue. Biopsy is not indicated unless there is any doubt of the initial diagnosis.

MANAGEMENT

In the past, treatment has consisted of topical antifungal therapy in the form of lozenges or pastilles, dissolved on the midline of the tongue 8-hourly for up to 3 months. Lack of patient compliance with this treatment may in part explain the poor therapeutic results. More recently, the use of systemic antifungal agents, such as fluconazole and itraconazole, has produced encouraging results.

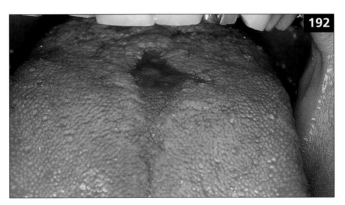

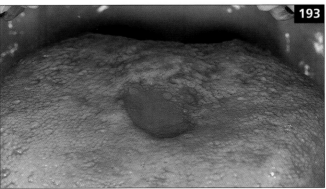

192, 193 Classic appearance of median rhomboid glossitis in the middle of the tongue.

Angular cheilitis

ETIOLOGY AND PATHOGENESIS
Angular cheilitis is often associated with the presence of intra-oral candidosis (candidiasis). Candida species can be isolated from approximately two-thirds of patients with angular cheilitis, either alone or in combination with staphylococci or streptococci. Colonization of the angles of the mouth with candida is probably a result of the direct spread of the organisms from the commensal oral microflora, while colonization with staphylococci is associated with the spread of bacteria from the chronic carriage of *Staphylococcus aureus* in the anterior nares.

CLINICAL FEATURES
This condition presents as erythema, possibly with yellow crusting at one or more (usually both) corners of the mouth (**194, 195**).

DIAGNOSIS
A separate smear or swab should be taken from each angle of the mouth, each side of the anterior nares, the palate and, if present, the fitting-surface of the upper denture. An oral rinse should be performed if no intra-oral appliance is present.

MANAGEMENT
Treatment is based on the eradication of the reservoir of candida in the mouth or staphylococci in the nose. Patients should apply a topical antimicrobial, such as miconazole that has activity against candida and staphylococci, every 6 hours. If appropriate, denture hygiene should be established. If staphylococci alone are isolated from both the angles and anterior nares, then fusidic acid or mupirocin should be prescribed for topical use 6-hourly. Two tubes of medication should be issued and the patient instructed to use one exclusively for the angles and the other for the anterior nares. Investigations for an underlying cause, such as diabetes or hematinic deficiency, should be undertaken if the angular cheilitis persists following local treatment.

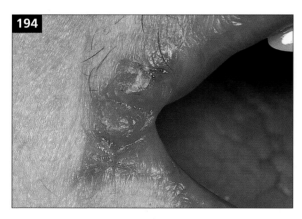

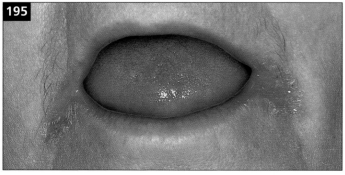

194, 195 Angular cheilitis presents as a reddening at the angles of the mouth. Gold crusting would suggest the presence of staphylococci rather than purely candidal infection.

Iron deficiency anemia

ETIOLOGY AND PATHOGENESIS

Iron deficiency anemia is the most frequent type of anemia and can occur in four settings: a decreased intake of iron, that occurs in starvation and malnutrition; a reduced absorption of iron due to intestinal disease; chronic loss of iron due to a gastrointestinal bleed; and an increased demand on iron requirements during pregnancy or childhood.

CLINICAL FEATURES

Iron deficiency anemia primarily affects females and presents clinically as lethargy, fatigue, pallor, and shortness of breath. Patients may have brittle, shovel-shaped nails (koilonychia) and brittle hair. Within the mouth, the oral mucosa may appear red, smooth, and is painful (**196**). Similar findings may also be seen as a component of the Plummer–Vinson syndrome in which iron deficiency anemia is accompanied by dysphagia, atrophy of the upper gastrointestinal mucosa, and a predisposition to oral cancer.

DIAGNOSIS

Diagnosis is suspected in the presence of typical clinical findings. Laboratory analysis of the blood shows hypochromic, microcytic anemia with reduced hemoglobin and a reduced hematocrit. Serum analysis will also show low iron levels and decreased serum ferritin but increased total iron binding capacity (transferrin).

MANAGEMENT

Management is primarily directed at determining and correcting the underlying cause of the iron deficiency. Dietary iron supplements can be used to replenish the iron stores although these should only be given once the etiology has been identified.

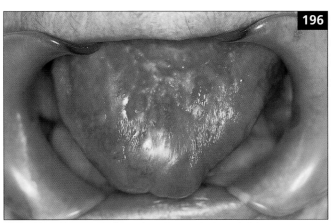

196 Atrophic and erythematous tongue in iron deficiency.

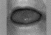

Pernicious anemia

ETIOLOGY AND PATHOGENESIS

Pernicious anemia is due to a deficiency of vitamin B_{12} which is necessary for DNA synthesis of rapidly dividing cells, such as those found in the bone marrow. The primary cause of pernicious anemia is auto-immune-mediated destruction of gastric parietal cells that produce intrinsic factor. Intrinsic factor binds to vitamin B_{12} in the stomach and is responsible for intestinal absorption of the vitamin. Much less frequently, pernicious anemia is due to dietary deficiency and only when there is a complete absence of meat and other animal products.

CLINICAL FEATURES

Patients have clinical signs and symptoms of anemia including weakness, lethargy, fatigue, shortness of breath, and pallor. In severe cases there are central neurologic manifestations, including peripheral neuropathies, headache, dizziness, and tinnitus. Within the mouth the dorsum of the tongue is erythematous, painful, and depapillated, so-called 'Hunter's glossitis' or 'Moeller's glossitis' (**197**). Angular cheilitis is also a presenting feature of pernicious anemia.

DIAGNOSIS

Examination of the peripheral blood shows a megaloblastic anemia, with an increased mean corpuscular volume (MCV). Serum vitamin B_{12} will be reduced. A Schilling test is often used to confirm a suspected diagnosis of pernicious anemia. This test consists of the oral administration of radioactive-labelled vitamin B_{12}, followed by a large flushing dose of non-radioactive vitamin B_{12} parenterally. The amount of radioactive-labelled vitamin B_{12} in the urine will be proportional to the amount of the orally administered vitamin B_{12} that is absorbed. Serum antibodies to gastric parietal cells are found in 90% of patients and antibodies to intrinsic factor in 60% of patients. These antibodies are also found in the saliva.

MANAGEMENT

The condition is managed by parenteral injections of vitamin B_{12} firstly on a weekly basis then subsequently at 1- or 3-monthly intervals for life. The oral symptoms of pernicious anemia resolve rapidly after the correction of the deficiency.

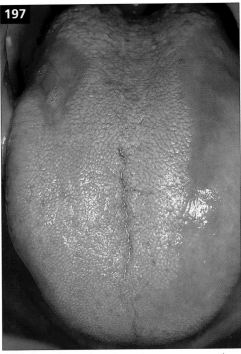

197 Atrophic and erythematous mucosa on the tongue in pernicious anemia.

Folic acid (folate) deficiency

ETIOLOGY AND PATHOGENESIS
Folic acid, like vitamin B_{12}, is essential for DNA synthesis and a deficiency results in a macrocytic anemia. The condition is similar to pernicious anemia but without the neurologic complications. The primary cause is malnutrition, overcooking of foods, alcoholism, small bowel disease, or pregnancy. Reduced levels of folic acid (folate) can also be seen as a complication of phenytoin or methotrexate therapy.

CLINICAL FEATURES
Patients with folic acid deficiency have symptoms of anemia including pallor, lethargy, fatigue, and shortness of breath. They may also suffer from diarrhea and other gastric abnormalities. Orally, the dorsum of the tongue is erythematous, painful, and depapillated (**198**). Angular cheilitis and recurrent aphthous stomatitis are other oral manifestations of folic acid (folate) deficiency.

DIAGNOSIS
Peripheral blood analysis will show megaloblastic, macrocytic anemia. There will be decreased serum and red cell folate levels. Urinary excretion of formiminoglutamic acid (FIGlu) is increased after the oral administration of histidine.

MANAGEMENT
Management is primarily directed at determining and subsequently correcting the cause of the folic acid (folate) deficiency. Replacement therapy with oral folic acid (folate), typically 5 mg daily, is then indicated. It is important to note that this therapy will correct the megaloblastic anemia of vitamin B_{12} deficiency but will not arrest the neurologic degeneration.

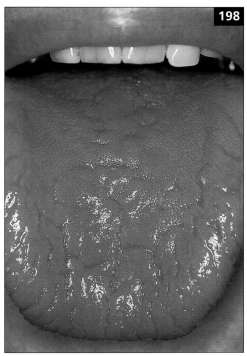

198 Atrophic tongue in folic acid (folate) deficiency.

Chronic erythematous (atrophic) candidosis (candidiasis)

ETIOLOGY AND PATHOGENESIS

This form of oral candidosis (candidiasis) is the most frequent, being present to some degree in the majority of patients who wear an upper denture. Continuous coverage of the palatal mucosa is a recognized predisposing factor for chronic erythematous candidosis (candidiasis). Colonization of the denture or other appliance results in inflammatory changes in the underlying mucosa.

CLINICAL FEATURES

The palatal mucosa is erythematous with margins corresponding to the periphery of the appliance worn. This condition is usually associated with full acrylic dentures (**199**) but may also occur under a partial denture (**200**) or an orthodontic appliance (**201**). In addition to being erythematous, the mucosa may also become nodular, a condition referred to as papillary hyperplasia (**202**).

DIAGNOSIS

A separate smear, swab, or imprint culture should be taken from the area of the affected mucosa and the fitting surface of the appliance. Although there may be minimal recovery of candida from the mucosa, the denture will be found to be heavily colonized.

MANAGEMENT

Ensuring adequate denture hygiene is the main principle of management of this infection. Daily mechanical cleaning of dentures is essential. In addition, the patient should be advised to place the prosthesis, if made of acrylic, in a dilute solution of hypochlorite overnight for 3 weeks. Patients who have a denture with metal components, such as cobalt chromium base or steel clasps, should soak the appliance in a 0.2% chlorhexidine solution. Placement of metal in hypochlorite will cause tarnishing. Topical polyene antifungal agents, such as amphotericin, nystatin, or miconazole, applied 6-hourly to the denture's fitting surface for 4 weeks will also speed the resolution of the condition.

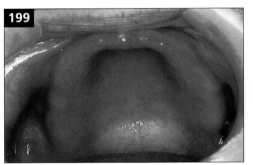

199 Erythematous candidosis (candidiasis) under a full denture.

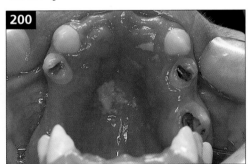

200 Erythematous candidosis (candidiasis) under a partial denture.

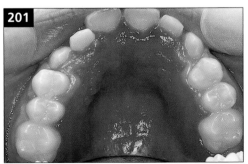

201 Erythematous candidosis (candidiasis) under an orthodontic appliance.

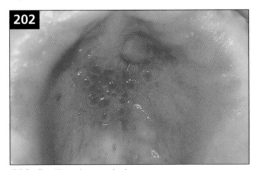

202 Papillary hyperplasia.

Erythroplakia

ETIOLOGY AND PATHOGENESIS

Erythroplakia is a clinical term used to describe 'a red patch or plaque on the oral mucosa that cannot be rubbed off and cannot be characterized clinically as any specific disease'. This definition therefore excludes conditions such as erosive lichen planus, geographic tongue, and erythematous candidosis (candidiasis). Most cases of erythroplakia are associated with a tobacco habit, although alcohol, invasive candidal infection, hematinic deficiency (Plummer–Vinson syndrome), and chronic trauma may also play a role. The malignant transformation rate of erythroplakia is between 5–10%.

CLINICAL FEATURES

Most cases of erythroplakia occur in the middle-aged and older populations. Any intra-oral site may be affected but the floor of the mouth is the most frequent (**203**). Clinically, erythroplakia may include white patches and is then referred to as 'speckled leukoplakia'.

DIAGNOSIS

A biopsy of an area of erythroplakia is mandatory since lesions with a similar clinical appearance have a range of differing histologic diagnoses, including carcinoma. In addition, it is essential to determine the severity of any epithelial dysplasia that may be present.

MANAGEMENT

In the absence of dysplasia, no treatment is required apart from periodic re-examination every 6 months to assess for clinical change that would indicate a need to re-biopsy. The management of lesions with dysplastic lesions will depend on the severity of the epithelial dysplasia. A mildly dysplastic leukoplakia may be managed conservatively with emphasis on the elimination of tobacco or alcohol habits, treatment of any candidal infection, and exclusion of any underlying hematinic deficiency. The provision of long-term retinoid therapy has been suggested to have a role in the management of mild dysplasia. However, recent evidence now shows that although retinoid therapy improves the clinical appearance of the lesions, genetic aberrations remain unaltered. Therefore, the efficacy of this therapy has been questioned. Re-biopsy should be performed after 3 months to assess the effect of measures aimed at the correction of etiologic factors. Long-term review at 6-monthly intervals is required. The role of exfoliative cytology and brush biopsy in monitoring such lesions is under review and may be helpful in the future. Although opinions do differ, severely dysplastic lesions should be managed as carcinoma due to the risk of malignant change. The role of photodynamic therapy in the management of localized severe dysplasia and small carcinoma is presently being evaluated.

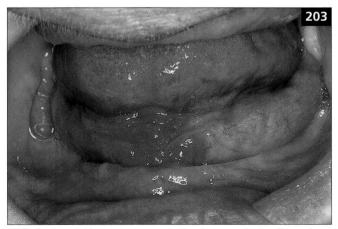

203 Erythroplakia seen as an area of red mucosa in the floor of the mouth.

Squamous cell carcinoma

ETIOLOGY AND PATHOGENESIS
The use of tobacco and alcohol remain the two most important risk factors associated with the development of oral squamous cell carcinoma (SCC) (Chapter 2, p. 28).

CLINICAL FEATURES
The clinical presentation of SCC is variable and ranges from a small area of erythema to a large swelling or ulcer. The most frequently affected intra-oral sites are the floor of the mouth (**204**), the tongue, and the retromolar region (**205, 206**).

DIAGNOSIS
Any erythematous area of mucosa should be viewed with suspicion and biopsy undertaken if there is doubt in diagnosis. Although a diagnosis of SCC can be suspected clinically the only method of definitive diagnosis is biopsy.

MANAGEMENT
The overall 5-year survival rate from oral SCC is approximately 40%. Management consists of surgery, radiotherapy, or a combination of both forms of treatment (Chapter 2, p. 28).

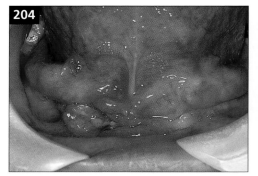

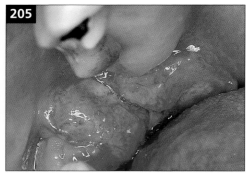

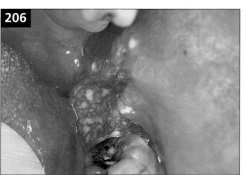

204–206 Squamous cell carcinoma presenting as an erythematous lesion in the floor of mouth and retromolar region. These are two sites frequently affected by oral cancer.

Infectious mononucleosis (glandular fever)

ETIOLOGY AND PATHOGENESIS

Infectious mononucleosis is caused by the Epstein–Barr virus, a herpes group member. EBV is transmitted in salivary droplets and initially infects B-lymphocytes. T-lymphocytes react to the infected B-cells and appear in the peripheral blood as atypical lymphocytes. Subsequently there is lymphoid proliferation in the blood, lymph nodes, and spleen.

CLINICAL FEATURES

The condition is characterized by lymph node enlargement, fever, and pharyngeal inflammation. Approximately 30% of patients will also suffer from purpura or petechiae in the palate and oral ulceration (**207**). Occasionally gingival bleeding and ulceration resembling acute necrotizing ulcerative gingivitis may develop. The condition occurs mainly in childhood or early adolescence.

DIAGNOSIS

Serologic demonstration of IgM antibody to Epstein–Barr virus capsid antigen and a positive Monospot slide test or Paul–Bunnell (Davidson) test will confirm a diagnosis of infectious mononucleosis.

MANAGEMENT

No specific treatment is required, although hospitalization may be necessary in severe cases of infectious mononucleosis with hepatic or splenic involvement. Ampicillin and its derivatives should be avoided since they are likely to produce an erythematous skin rash.

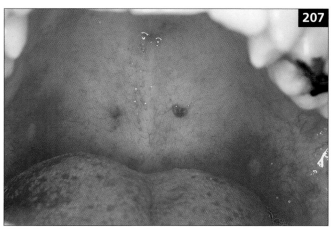

207 Petechiae and ulcers in the palate associated with infectious mononucleosis.

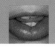

Swelling

- **General approach**
- **Bacterial sialadenitis**
- **Viral sialadenitis (mumps)**
- **Sialosis (sialadenosis)**
- **Mucocoele and ranula**
- **Salivary gland tumor (major gland)**
- **Squamous cell carcinoma**
- **Crohn's disease**
- **Orofacial granulomatosis**
- **Paget's disease (osteitis deformans)**
- **Acromegaly**
- **Fibroepithelial polyp (focal fibrous hyperplasia, irritation fibroma)**
- **Drug-induced gingival hyperplasia**
- **Focal epithelial hyperplasia (Heck's disease)**
- **Salivary gland tumor (minor gland)**
- **Denture-induced hyperplasia (denture granuloma)**
- **Pyogenic granuloma (pregnancy epulis)**
- **Peripheral giant cell granuloma (giant cell epulis)**
- **Squamous papilloma**
- **Infective warts (verruca vulgaris, condylomata acuminata)**
- **Bone exostosis**
- **Sialolith (salivary stone)**
- **Tongue piercing**
- **Lymphoma**

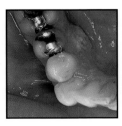
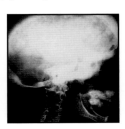
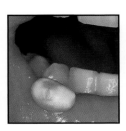
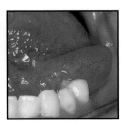

General approach

- Swelling of the orofacial tissues may be due to trauma, infection, immune reactions, or neoplasia.
- Chronic swellings of the oral tissues are usually painless.
- Swelling may be extra-oral, intra-oral, or at both sites.
- Differentiation of intra-oral swelling may be achieved on the basis of the presence of ulceration and the color of the lesion.

The causes of extra- and intra-oral swelling are given in *Tables* 5 and 6.

Table 5 Causes of extra-oral swelling

- Suppurative sialadenitis
- Viral sialadenitis
- Sialosis
- Ranula
- Salivary gland tumor
- Squamous cell carcinoma
- Crohn's disease
- Orofacial granulomatosis
- Paget's disease
- Fibrous dysplasia
- Acromegaly

Table 6 Causes of intra-oral swelling

Pink
- Fibroepithelial polyp
- Drug-induced hyperplasia
- Warts and condylomata
- Focal epithelial hyperplasia
- Crohn's disease
- Orofacial granulomatosis
- Squamous cell carcinoma
- Salivary gland tumor

Red
- Denture-induced hyperplasia
- Pyogenic granuloma
- Giant cell granuloma
- Squamous cell carcinoma
- Scurvy

White
- Squamous papilloma
- Squamous cell carcinoma

Blue
- Mucocele
- Ranula

Yellow
- Sialolith
- Bone exostosis

Bacterial sialadenitis

ETIOLOGY AND PATHOGENESIS
Any cause of reduced salivary flow can permit the retrograde infection of a major salivary gland with members of the commensal oral microflora. Dehydration following major surgery was formerly an important predisposing factor for bacterial sialadenitis, but improved understanding of fluid balance has almost eliminated this complication. Traditionally, the microorganisms encountered in this infection have been *Staphylocoocus aureus*, *Streptococcus viridans*, and *Streptococcus pneumoniae*. However, more recently it has become apparent that strictly anerobic bacteria are also involved.

CLINICAL FEATURES
The affected gland is painful, swollen (**208**), and tender to touch with a purulent discharge from the duct orifice (**209, 210**). The overlying skin may be erythematous and the patient will have fever and malaise.

DIAGNOSIS
Diagnosis is made based on the history and clinical findings. Rarely, a child may be found to have suffered repeated episodes of acute sialadenitis in one parotid gland, a condition known as recurrent parotitis of childhood (**211**). This unusual diagnosis can be confirmed by sialography that will show multiple sialectasis within the parotid gland (**212**).

MANAGEMENT

Management should consist of empirical antibiotic therapy with cloxacillin, amoxicillin (amoxycillin) or metronidazole. If possible a sample of pus should be collected from the duct orifice by aspiration. In the acute phase the patient will gain pain relief from the provision of a nonsteroidal anti-inflammatory drug. A dehydrated patient should be rehydrated and the fluid balance established. Once the acute symptoms have resolved, a sialogram should be performed to determine the presence of any structural abnormality within the affected gland.

Each episode of infection in the situation of recurrent parotitis of childhood should be managed individually. Interestingly, this rare condition resolves after puberty.

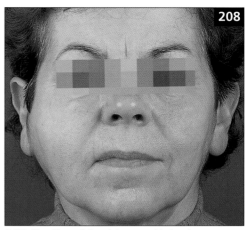

208 Swelling of the right parotid gland.

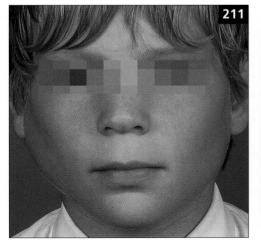

209 Purulent discharge from the parotid duct orifice.

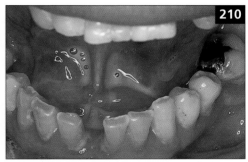

210 Pus draining from the left submandibular gland duct orifice into the floor of the mouth.

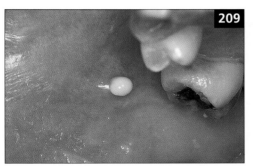

211 Swelling of the left parotid gland of a boy with recurrent parotitis of childhood.

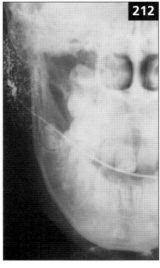

212 Sialogram showing multiple sialectais characteristic of recurrent parotitis of childhood.

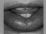

Viral sialadenitis (mumps)

ETIOLOGY AND PATHOGENESIS

Mumps represents an acute viral sialadenitis predominantly involving the parotid glands, although other glands may be affected. Infection is caused by a paramyxovirus that is highly infectious and transmitted by saliva. A 2–3 week incubation period precedes the clinical symptoms.

CLINICAL FEATURES

Mumps mostly occurs in childhood but may occasionally develop in adults. The principal manifestations are fever, malaise, headache, chills, and pre-auricular pain with swelling. Approximately 75% of patients have bilateral parotid gland disease (**213**). The swelling is maximal 2–3 days after the onset of clinical symptoms, with most of the swelling disappearing 10 days later. Since mumps is a systemic infection other organs can be involved, including the gonads, liver, pancreas, and kidneys. Orchitis and oophoritis in adulthood is a serious complication since it can lead to sterility.

DIAGNOSIS

Most cases can be diagnosed on a clinical basis. When there is doubt the diagnosis can be confirmed by the demonstration of raised serum antibodies to S and V antigens of the paramyxovirus. Antibody to the S antigen disappears shortly after infection but antibody to V antigen persists and may be used as a marker of previous infection. The virus can also be cultured from the saliva.

MANAGEMENT

Treatment is symptomatic consisting of rest, fluids, and analgesia (acetaminophen [paracetamol]). Aspirin is not recommended in children. Adults who develop gonad involvement should be given in the region of 40 mg of oral prednisolone (prednisone) daily for 4 days, which is then gradually reduced.

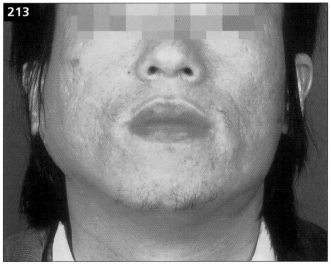

213 Bilateral swelling of the parotid glands in mumps.

Sialosis (sialadenosis)

ETIOLGY AND PATHOGENESIS

This condition represents a noninflammatory, non-neoplastic swelling of the major salivary glands, principally the parotid glands. The etiology is poorly understood, although a number of conditions have been implicated in the possible cause. Factors associated with sialosis include alcoholic abuse, cirrhosis, diabetes, anorexia, and bulimia.

CLINICAL FEATURES

Sialosis presents with a painless bilateral enlargement of the parotid glands (**214**).

DIAGNOSIS

Diagnosis is made on the clinical findings and history. Biospy is not required, although if undertaken reveals hypertrophy of the serous acini and edema of the interstitial connective tissue. Hematologic investigations should be undertaken to exclude other causes of chronic swelling of the parotid glands.

MANAGEMENT

Once diagnosed no active treatment is required.

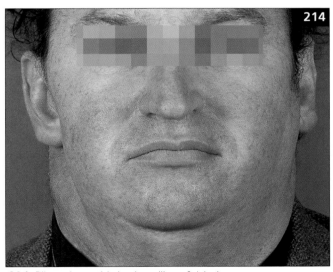

214 Bilateral parotid gland swelling of sialosis.

Mucocele and ranula

ETIOLOGY AND PATHOGENESIS

An accumulation of mucus either in the connective tissues or within a salivary duct is clinically termed a mucocele (Chapter 3, p. 48) and encompasses both mucous extravasation phenomenon and mucus retention cysts. The mucous extravasation phenomenon is the result of trauma or transection of a salivary duct, leading to mucous spillage into the connective tissues with resultant granulation tissue response. A mucous retention cyst may be the result of duct obstruction secondary to a salivary stone, scarring, or an adjacent tumor.

CLINICAL FEATURES

Mucocele may develop at any oral site but presents most frequently as a bluish fluid-filled sessile mass just below the mucosa of the lower lip. Blockage of the submandibular or sublingual gland duct may cause a large mucocele in the floor of the mouth, with external swelling. Such a mucocele is sometimes termed a ranula after a suggested resemblance to a frog's belly and the Latin term for frog (**215, 216**). A plunging ranula is the result of herniation of the lesion through the mylohyoid muscle and along the fascial planes of the neck. These can present as midline masses in the neck and rarely in the mediastinum.

DIAGNOSIS

Diagnosis of mucocele is made on the history and examination. Excisional biopsy including the adjacent minor salivary glands is curative and diagnosis of either extravasation or retention is confirmed by the histopathological findings. Imaging using ultrasound, CT, or MRI of the floor of the mouth and the neck may be needed to determine the extent of a ranula.

MANAGEMENT

Mucoceles are treated by surgical excision to include the lesion and the adjacent minor salivary glands. Aspiration produces no lasting benefit since the adjacent salivary glands will quickly refill the mucocele. The surgical site is frequently left to heal by secondary intention to minimize the chance of recurrence. Cryotherapy may be used to treat mucoceles in children, although there is a possibility of recurrence.

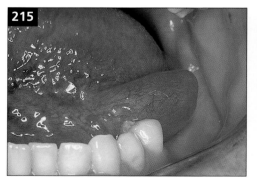

215 Mucocele in the floor of the mouth.

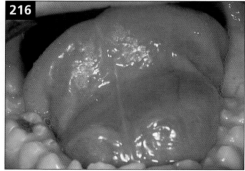

216 Large mucocele (ranula) in the floor of the mouth.

Salivary gland tumor (major gland)

ETIOLOGY AND PATHOGENESIS

There are a number of types of salivary gland tumor, all of which are relatively rare and usually present as swelling. The majority (85%) of salivary tumors affect the major glands, with almost 90% of these arising in the parotid gland. The main types of tumor include pleomorphic adenoma, papillary cystadenoma lymphomatosum (Warthin tumor), mucoepidermoid carcinoma, acinic cell carcinoma, adenoid cystic carcinoma, and polymorphous low-grade adenocarcinoma. The exact diagnosis of a salivary tumor can only be made after biopsy.

Pleomorphic salivary adenoma (PSA) is a benign tumor and the most common neoplasm of both the major and minor salivary glands. Approximately 75% of all tumors arising in the parotid gland are PSA. The etiology is unknown but pathologic features suggest that it is derived from the neoplastic transformation of salivary ductal and myoepithelial cells.

CLINICAL FEATURES

PSA presents as a firm, lobulated mass either extra-orally within a major gland (**217**) or intra-orally from minor gland tissue (**218**). The overlying mucosa or skin appears similar to the adjacent tissues. Lesions are slow-growing and painless, ranging in size from a few millimeters to several centimeters. Within the mouth, the majority of these tumors are located in the palate, the buccal mucosa, or the upper lip.

DIAGNOSIS

Diagnosis is established on the histopathologic examination of biopsy material that will show bilayered duct structures composed of neoplastic acinar cells variably mixed with myoepthelial cells and a stroma ranging from hyaline material to cartilage and bone. Imaging studies, such as ultrasound, CT, or MRI are often necessary to determine the extent of the disease, particularly when PSA occurs within a major salivary gland.

MANAGEMENT

Surgical excision is the treatment of choice. Enucleation is not an acceptable therapy since small fingers of tumor that are located within and outside the tumor capsule are left behind and contribute to recurrence. Incomplete excision is the most important factor related to tumor recurrence. Malignant change, referred to as carcinoma ex-PSA, can occasionally occur in untreated PSA.

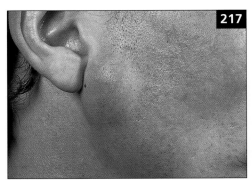

217 Pleomorphic salivary adenoma in the parotid gland.

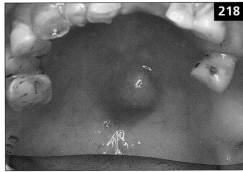

218 Pleomorphic salivary adenoma in the palate.

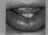

Squamous cell carcinoma

ETIOLOGY AND PATHOGENESIS

The use of tobacco and alcohol remain the two most important risk factors associated with the development of oral squamous cell carcinoma (SCC) (Chapter 2, p. 28).

CLINICAL FEATURES

SCC has no characteristic appearance and can present with a variety of clinical signs including swelling, white patch (Chapter 4, p. 76), red patch (Chapter 5, p. 94), or ulceration (Chapter 2, p. 28). Fixation to underlying tissues is a feature common to all forms. A large SCC within the mouth may produce obvious extra-oral swelling (**219**). If metastasis has occurred then the regional lymph nodes may be palpable or visibly enlarged (**220**). SCC of the lip can present as a firm swelling that is palpable within the tissues (**221**). Intra-orally SCC can develop as a swelling at any site, although most frequently in the floor of the mouth (**222**, **223**), the tongue, and the retro-molar region (**224**). The gingivae (**225**, **226**) and the buccal mucosa (**227**) are relatively rare sites for SCC.

DIAGNOSIS

Diagnosis is made on examination of material from an incisional biopsy. Small suspicious lesions should be excised at the time of the initial biopsy.

MANAGEMENT

Treatment consists of surgery, radiotherapy, or a combination of approaches. Chemotherapy has a limited role in management of SCC (Chapter 2, p. 28).

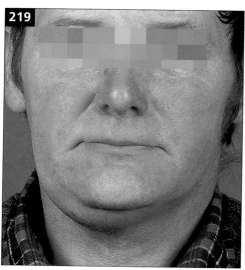

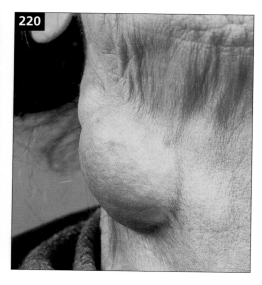

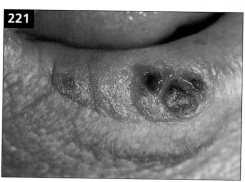

219 Right submandibular swelling due to a large squamous cell carcinoma in the floor of the mouth.

220 Lymph node swelling due to the metastasis of squamous cell carcinoma from the floor of the mouth and tongue.

221 Squamous cell carcinoma presenting as swelling of the lower lip. A visible lesion such as this is often detected while small, in contrast to intra-oral lesions which are frequently not diagnosed until relatively large.

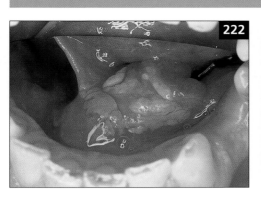

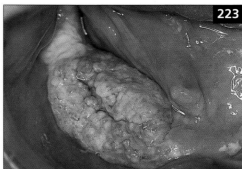

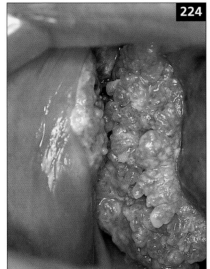

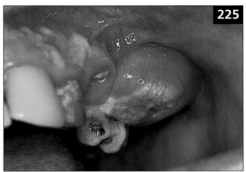

222–227 Squamous cell carcinoma presenting as swelling at various oral sites.

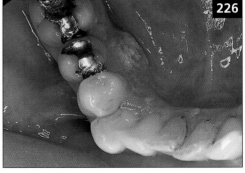

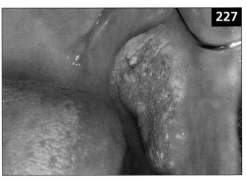

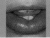

Crohn's disease

ETIOLOGY AND PATHOGENESIS
Crohn's disease is a nonspecific inflammatory bowel disease of unknown etiology that can affect any portion of the gastrointestinal tract from the mouth to the anus. The prevalence in the population is 2–6/100,000. The condition is more common in Jews than in Asians or blacks. Genetic factors are likely to play a role in its development since 10–15% of affected patients have a first-degree relative with either Crohn's disease or ulcerative colitis. There is also a high concordance in monozygotic twins.

CLINICAL FEATURES
Inflammation of the small intestine may impair the absorption of vital nutrients. Iron and folate are absorbed in the duodenum while vitamin B_{12} is absorbed from the terminal ileum. Disease at these sites may therefore result in deficiencies that are detectable in peripheral blood. In addition, poor absorptive function of the small bowel is likely to result in low albumin levels.

Gastrointestinal symptoms are the predominant finding with pain, diarrhea, cramping, fever, and weight loss. One-third of sufferers have orofacial signs and symptoms at the time of the initial presentation. The oral manifestations are varied but typically there is diffuse perioral lip swelling (**228**), a nodular buccal mucosa with a cobblestone appearance (**229**), and mucosal tags (**230**). Ulceration that resembles recurrent aphthous stomatitis may also be present.

DIAGNOSIS
Diagnosis is made on clinical examination supplemented with biopsy of oral lesions that show non-caseating granulomatous inflammation with Langhans-type giant cells. Serology shows an elevated erythrocyte sedimentation rate, leukocytosis, and abnormal liver function tests. Ileo-colonoscopy with biopsy may be necessary.

MANAGEMENT
Sulfasalazine (sulphasalazine) is the main form of treatment to control the disease and oral symptoms will respond to the successful treatment of the intestinal involvement. In severe cases or an episode of acute symptoms, systemic steroids may also be used. Surgery is reserved for cases of intestinal fibrosis and fistulae.

Management of a patient with Crohn's disease should include regular review to monitor health of the oral soft tissues and level of dental caries. Topical steroid therapy can help reduce oral symptoms of ulceration. Antimicrobial agents are often required to treat secondary oral candidosis (candidiasis) or staphylococcal infection, which may present as angular cheilitis.

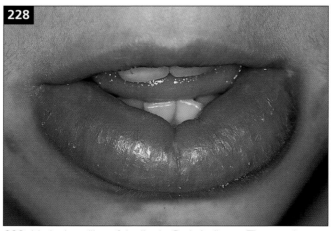

228 Marked swelling of the lips in Crohn's disease. The severity of swelling can vary considerably but often reflects the degree of underlying bowel activity.

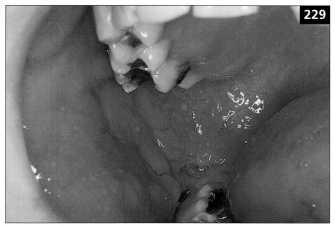

229 Cobblestone appearance in the buccal mucosa in Crohn's disease.

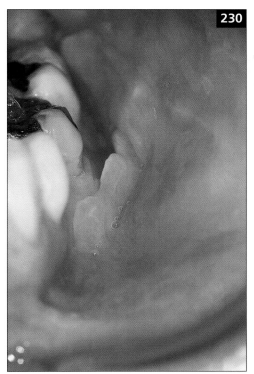

230 Mucosal tags in the lower buccal sulcus in Crohn's disease.

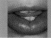

Orofacial granulomatosis

ETIOLOGY AND PATHOGENESIS

As evident from the name, this condition is characterized by granulomatous inflammation in the orofacial region. The cause of orofacial granulomatosis is not known. Infection with atypical mycobacteria has been suggested but not proven. A hypersensitivity to foodstuffs, in particular benzoic acid and cinnamon, has been implicated in the development of clinical symptoms.

CLINICAL FEATURES

This condition principally presents in childhood. The lips are the tissues most frequently affected, showing diffuse enlargement (**231**). Either lip or both can be affected. When facial swelling is accompanied by facial palsy and a fissure tongue the condition is termed Melkerson–Rosenthal syndrome, although few patients ever have the complete triad. Intra-oral features include a full thickness gingivitis (**232–234**), mucosal tags or folds in the buccal sulcus, and a cobblestone appearance of the buccal mucosa. There is often a history of atopic disease, such as childhood eczema or asthma.

DIAGNOSIS

Diagnosis is made on the basis of clinical presentation and biopsy of the buccal mucosa to reveal non-caseating granulomas. The buccal mucosa is a preferable site to the lip due to the likelihood of extreme swelling if the lip was subjected to a biopsy. Special stains for acid-fast bacilli are negative and there is no evidence of foreign material in the granulomata. Hematological investigations are normal with no evidence of an elevated erythrocyte sedimentation rate (ESR) or abnormalities of calcium, albumen, and folic acid (folate). Serum levels of angiotensin converting enzyme (ACE) will be normal, in contrast to sarcoidosis where levels are elevated. A normal neutrophil nitroblue tetrazolium reduction test will exclude a diagnosis of chronic granulomatous disease. A radio-allergen sorbent test (RAST) may show raised levels of IgE.

MANAGEMENT

Intra-lesional steroids may lead to a reduction of the soft tissue swelling but the effect is short-lived and repeated injections are frequently necessary. Cutaneous patch testing often reveals a hypersensitivity to benzoic acid, benzoates (E210–E219), cinnamon, and chocolate. Symptomatic improvement occurs if the patient is provided with appropriate advice on dietary exclusion from a dietician (**235, 236**), although strict avoidance is required.

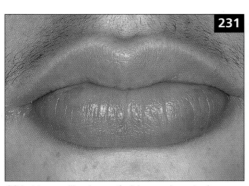

231 Lip swelling in orofacial granulomatosis.

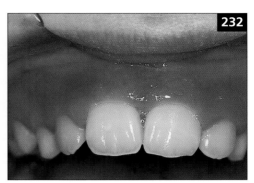

232 Full thickness gingivitis orofacial granulomatosis.

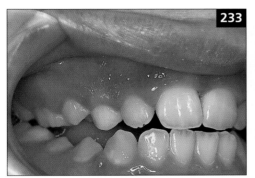

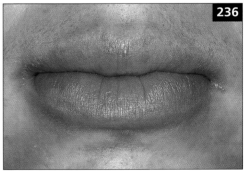

233, 234 Full thickness gingivitis orofacial granulomatosis.

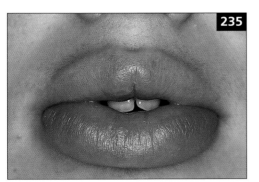

235 Lips of a patient with orofacial granulomatosis before the exclusion of benzoates from the diet.

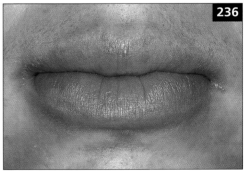

236 Lips of a patient with orofacial granulomatosis after the exclusion of benzoates from the diet.

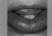

Paget's disease (osteitis deformans)

ETIOLOGY AND PATHOGENESIS

Paget's disease is a chronic, slowly progressive disorder of bone metabolism with no known etiology. The disease is characterized by excessive resorption and deposition of bone. Several theories have been proposed for Paget's disease including auto-immunity, an endocrine abnormality, autonomic nervous system–vascular disorder, and paramyxovirus infection of osteoclasts, but none of these have been proven.

CLINICAL FEATURES

Paget's disease is characterized by the progressive enlargement of the maxilla and mandible (**237**). The condition affects older patients, with 3–4% of middle-aged individuals and 10–15% of the elderly having some degree of Paget's disease. There is a strong family history in 15% of patients and it is more common in individuals of North European descent. The maxilla is affected more than the mandible, although in about 20% of cases there is involvement of both maxilla and mandible. Edentulous patients will complain of dentures that are too tight to wear and, if the cranium is involved, that their hat size has increased. Bone pain, headache, auditory and visual disturbances reflect the compression of neurovascular elements within narrowing foramina of the skull.

DIAGNOSIS

Diagnosis is established on the radiographic appearance of dense new bone in a 'cotton wool' pattern (**238**). Serum studies will show a strikingly elevated alkaline phosphatase but normal calcium and phosphate levels. There will also be elevated urinary hydroxyproline and calcium levels. Radiographs are likely to reveal hypercementosis and ankylosis of the teeth (**239, 240**).

MANAGEMENT

Paget's disease is essentially incurable. Calcitonin and biphosphonates can be used to control the excessive osteoclastic activity that characterizes the condition. Extraction of teeth is likely to be complicated and will need to involve a surgical approach.

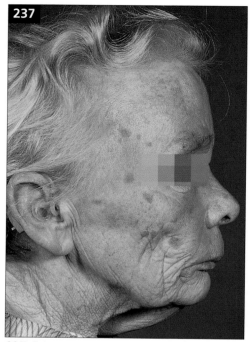

237 Enlargement of the skull and maxilla in Paget's disease.

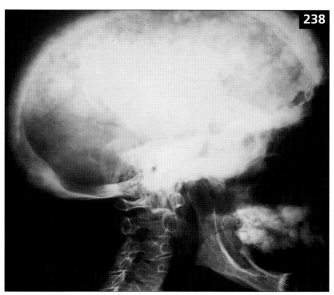

238 Lateral skull radiograph showing generalized radio-opacity of the calvarium and maxilla.

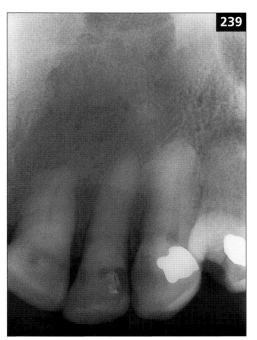

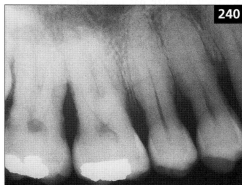

239, 240 Periapical radiographs showing hyper-cementosis and ankylosis of the upper teeth.

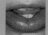

Acromegaly

ETIOLOGY AND PATHOGENESIS

Acromegaly is a rare condition caused by the hypersecretion of growth hormone from a pituitary adenoma in adulthood. The amount of growth hormone that is produced is proportional to the size of the pituitary adenoma. If hypersecretion of growth hormone occurs before closure of the epiphyseal plates in childhood then gigantism is the result.

CLINICAL FEATURES

Acromegaly is most often seen in the fourth decade of life. The condition and its manifestations develop slowly. Signs and symptoms include weakness, paresthesia, hypertension, and cardiac disease. Classically, there is enlargement of the maxilla and mandible (241) with separation of the teeth (242) and the development of a posterior cross-bite. The soft tissues, including the lips and the skin of the face, become thickened and appear coarse.

DIAGNOSIS

Diagnosis is made by the radiographic demonstration of an enlarged pituitary gland in the sella turcica. Serum levels of growth hormone are elevated.

MANAGEMENT

Acromegaly is managed by trans-sphenoidal removal of the pituitary adenoma. Radiotherapy is also occasionally used and is effective in reducing the size of the pituitary adenoma. Bromocriptine, a dopamine agonist, or octreotide are used as an adjunct to surgery or radiotherapy but not as primary therapy.

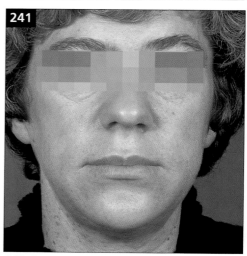

241 Enlargement of the mandible due to acromegaly.

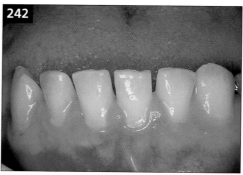

242 Spacing of the teeth due to acromegaly.

Fibroepithelial polyp (focal fibrous hyperplasia, irritation fibroma)

ETIOLOGY AND PATHOGENESIS

The etiology of a fibroepithelial polyp is unknown but it is likely that chronic minor irritation plays a role.

CLINICAL FEATURES

Classically fibroepithelial polyp presents as a single, rubbery, sessile or pedunculated, painless swelling with normal overlying mucosa or a slightly keratotic surface. Any intra-oral site can be affected but most commonly they arise on the labial mucosa, tongue, and buccal mucosa at the occlusal line (**243–246**).

DIAGNOSIS

Although diagnosis of a fibroepithelial polyp can frequently be made on clinical examination alone, surgical removal is the treatment of choice and therefore clinical diagnosis can be confirmed histopathologically.

MANAGEMENT

Fibroepithelial polyps should be treated by surgical excision. To reduce the likelihood of recurrence, any source of irritation should be corrected.

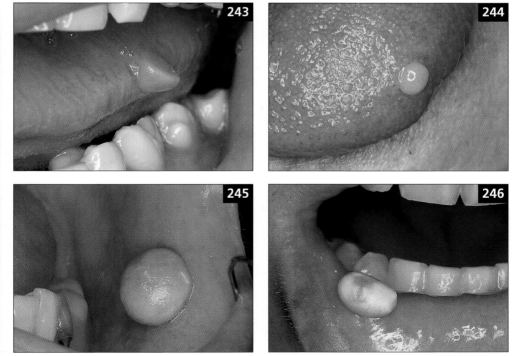

243–246 Swelling of fibroepithelial polyp, with characteristic smooth surface, at various oral sites.

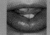

Drug-induced gingival hyperplasia

ETIOLOGY AND PATHOGENESIS
A number of drugs are known to have an adverse effect of causing gingival hyperplasia. Phenytoin, an anti-seizure medication, is the most widely recognized medication associated with fibrous overgrowth of the gingival tissues, occurring in approximately 50% of patients taking the drug. The hyperplasia is believed to be due to the alteration of collagen metabolism by gingival fibroblasts. Calcium channel blockers and the immunosuppressive ciclosporin (cyclosporin) also cause gingival hyerplasia in 10–20 % of patients. In addition, mild hyperplasia is a recognized phenomenon with oral contraceptives.

CLINICAL FEATURES
There is increased bulk of the free and attached gingivae, particularly the inter-dental papillae (247, 248). In phenytoin-induced hyperplasia, the gingivae appears pink, firm and rubbery, reflecting the enhanced collagen content. For calcium channel blockers and ciclosporin (cyclosporin), the appearance of the enlargement ranges in color from red to pink and in consistency from firm to spongy.

DIAGNOSIS
Diagnosis is based on the clinical presentation and a history of use of a drug reported to produce hyperplasia. Biopsy is nonspecific apart from lesions induced by phenytoin which contain strikingly dense collagen and entrapped islands of epithelium.

MANAGEMENT
In all cases oral hygiene needs to be optimal since inflammation appears to precipitate or even worsen the hyperplasia. Gingivoplasty is frequently necessary to treat gingival hyperplasia, particularly those induced by phenytoin, although some regression can be expected if the calcium channel blocker, ciclosporin (cyclosporin), or oral contraceptive is discontinued.

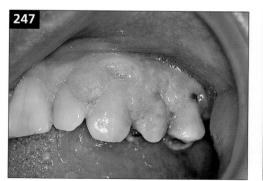
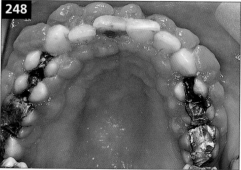

247, 248 Drug-induced gingival hyperplasia.

Focal epithelial hyperplasia (Heck's disease)

ETIOLOGY AND PATHOGENESIS
This is a benign condition first described in Native Americans and the Inuit, but also now seen in other populations. An infectious etiology due to human papilloma viruses (HPV types 13 and 32) has been shown by both epidemiologic and molecular studies.

CLINICAL FEATURES
The lesions appear as discrete or clustered, smooth-topped, pink papules, most frequently on the buccal mucosa, labial mucosa, tongue (**249**), and gingivae. The papules are asymptomatic.

DIAGNOSIS
Diagnosis is made on examination of biopsy material that will reveal an acanthotic, hyperkeratotic epithelium containing vacuolated prickle cells. Ultrastructural studies will show 50 nm viral particles of HPV.

MANAGEMENT
No treatment may be needed for asymptomatic cases. For more widespread lesions surgical excision using cautery or laser may be necessary. It has been noted that some cases of focal epithelial hyperplasia undergo spontaneous regression.

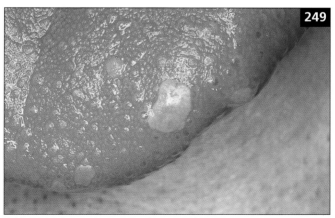

249 Multiple papules on the dorsum of the tongue in Heck's disease.

Salivary gland tumor (minor gland)

There are a number of types of salivary gland tumor, all of which are relatively rare and usually present as swelling. The majority (85%) of salivary tumors affect the major glands, with almost 90% of these arising in the parotid gland. The main types of tumor include pleomorphic adenoma, papillary cystadenoma lymphomatosum (Warthin tumor), mucoepidermoid carcinoma, acinic cell carcinoma, adenoid cystic carcinoma, and polymorphous low-grade adenocarcinoma. While adenoid cystic carcinoma accounts for only 25% of carcinomas occurring in the salivary glands, this type of tumor comprises the majority (50–70%) of all neoplasms arising in the minor salivary glands.

ETIOLOGY AND PATHOGENESIS
The cause of adenoid cystic carcinoma is not known. Pathologic features suggest that adenoid cystic carcinoma is derived from the neoplastic transformation of myoepithelial cells.

CLINICAL FEATURES
Within the mouth, adenoid cystic carcinoma presents most frequently as a firm, painless swelling in the palate (**250, 251**), possibly with superficial ulceration. When adenoid cystic carcinoma develops in the parotid gland, the fixed discrete swelling is often associated with facial nerve palsy.

DIAGNOSIS
Diagnosis is established by biopsy. Once diagnosed, imaging studies involving CT scan or MRI are required to determine the extent of the tumor. In the case of large lesions in major glands, such imaging or ultra-sound is likely to be performed prior to the biopsy.

MANAGEMENT
Adenoid cystic carcinoma is notoriously difficult to treat successfully. Surgery involving a wide margin is the treatment of choice. In the parotid gland, parotidectomy is performed with the sacrifice of the facial nerve if involved. Postoperative radiotherapy may be used in some situations. Chemotherapy plays little or no role in the management of this condition. The 5-year survival rate is about 70%, although the 15-year survival rate is only 10%. This outcome probably reflects the slow but relentlessly infiltrative growth and perineural spread of this tumor.

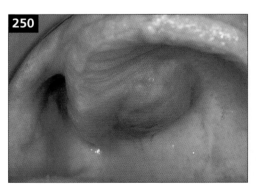

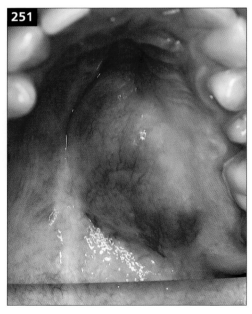

250, 251 Swelling of the palatal tissues due to adenoid cystic carcinoma. The overlying mucosa is normal suggesting that the origin of the lesion is within the underlying tissues.

Denture-induced hyperplasia (denture granuloma)

ETIOLOGY AND PATHOGENESIS

Denture-induced hyperplasia develops as a result of chronic irritation from the periphery of over-extended or poorly-fitting dentures. Excess collagen is produced, resulting in multiple submucosal masses.

CLINICAL FEATURES

This condition typically presents as painless, pink, lobulated masses in the mandibular (**252**) or maxillary (**253**) vestibules or palate (**254**). Ulceration often develops in the base of the folds, where the denture flange abuts. The appearance can be of concern, both to the clinician and the patient, due to the similarity to squamous cell carcinoma. Occasionally, there may be a single pedunculated lesion in the palate (**255**).

DIAGNOSIS

Diagnosis is made on the clinical appearance and is confirmed by examination of excised tissue that shows a dense fibrous tissue covered by hyperplastic epithelium.

MANAGEMENT

In almost all cases the hyperplastic tissue requires excision. Some reduction will occur in the short term if the denture flange is reduced. However, the mass is composed of dense scar tissue and will not regress significantly even if the denture is modified. Once the tissue is excised, a new denture can be made.

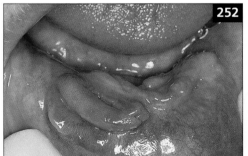
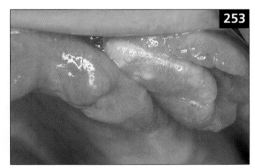
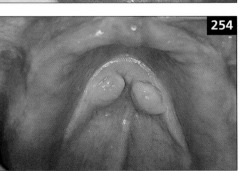
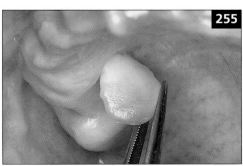

252–254 Tissue folds in regions corresponding to the edges of the denture (denture-induced hyperplasia).

255 Pedunculated hyperplasia ('leaf fibroma').

Pyogenic granuloma (pregnancy epulis)

ETIOLOGY AND PATHOGENESIS
Pyogenic granuloma is an exuberant growth of granulation tissue in response to trauma or irritation from factors such as calculus or a foreign body. Poor oral hygiene is also a well recognized predisposing factor. However, a predisposing factor is rarely identified. An exception to this is the hormonal change during pregnancy that in part contributes to the development of pyogenic granuloma; hence the term 'pregnancy epulis' in this situation.

CLINICAL FEATURES
Pyogenic granuloma appears as a nodular red lesion that is ulcerated and bleeds easily on touch (256–258). This lesion can occur at any site but frequently arises on the gingival margin.

DIAGNOSIS
A periapical radiograph should be taken to determine if there has been any underlying bone resorption. The diagnosis is confirmed by excisional biopsy showing a nodule of loose connective tissue containing many blood vessels and a dense inflammatory infiltrate.

MANAGEMENT
Pyogenic granuloma should be removed surgically. Any obvious irritant should be eliminated. In the case of a pregnant patient, small lesions may be left untreated since many will regress post-partum. Larger lesions and those that bleed frequently can be excised under local anesthesia. Recurrences occasionally occur and are typically related to continued trauma, persistent irritation, or poor oral hygiene.

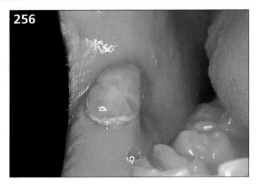

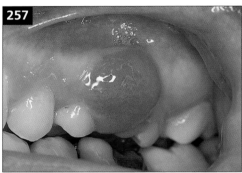

256, 257 Pyogenic granuloma. Note the ulcerated and vascular nature of this lesion, which differentiates it from the smooth, pink appearance of fibroepithelial polyp.

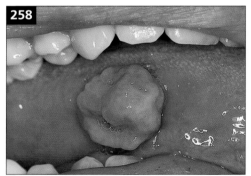

258 Pyogenic granuloma in a pregnant patient (pregnancy epulis).

Peripheral giant cell granuloma (giant cell epulis)

ETIOLOGY AND PATHOGENESIS
This is an uncommon hyperplastic connective tissue response to injury. Peripheral giant cell granuloma is thought to have similar etiology to pyogenic granuloma but histologically the lesion contains numerous foreign body-type giant cells.

CLINICAL FEATURES
This lesion characteristically presents appears as a red to blue mass that may be ulcerated, on the gingivae anterior to the first molar teeth (**259**). Resorption of the underlying alveolar bone can be seen radiographically, although this is not extensive.

DIAGNOSIS
Clinically the lesion is indistinguishable from a pyogenic granuloma and differentiation can only be made on the basis of histopathologic findings. Giant cell granuloma comprises a nodule of cellular mesenchyme filled with numerous giant cells. Serologic tests for levels of calcium, phosphate, and parathyroid hormone are advisable to exclude hyperparathyroidism. It is important to exclude, by radiography, the presence of a central giant cell granuloma that may have undergone extension into the soft tissues.

MANAGEMENT
The lesion should be excised surgically and any irritant removed.

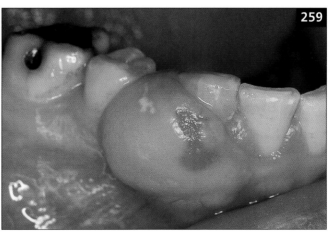

259 Peripheral giant cell granuloma.

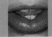

Squamous papilloma

ETIOLOGY AND PATHOGENESIS
The cause of squamous papilloma is unknown, but the involvement of human papillomavirus (HPV) has been suggested. Support for a viral cause is provided by the similarity in clinical appearance to the common wart (verruca vulgaris) occurring on the skin. The route of transmission, if viral, is not known but is likely to be due to direct contact.

CLINICAL FEATURES
The most frequent site of involvement is the labial mucosa, soft and hard palate, uvula, and lingual frenum. Squamous papilloma is typically a relatively small lesion with a white, granular surface producing a 'cauliflower-like' appearance (260–262). The lesions are usually solitary, but multiple lesions can occur.

DIAGNOSIS
The clinical appearance is characteristic but most lesions are removed and therefore histopathologic findings can confirm the diagnosis.

MANAGEMENT
Excision is usually curative and recurrence is uncommon except in immunocompromised individuals.

Infective warts (verruca vulgaris, condylomata acuminata)

ETIOLOGY AND PATHOGENESIS
Over 70 types of human papillomavirus (HPV) have been described and a number of these have been implicated in lesions of the oral mucosa. Intra-oral verruca vulgaris usually develops as a result of transmission of infection involving HPV types 2 and 4 from warts on the hands or fingers (263). Alternatively, oral lesions may arise due to direct oral contact with condyloma acuminata (venereal warts) (264) caused by HPV types 6, 11, and 60. HIV infection has been associated with a predisposition to multiple oral warts.

CLINICAL FEATURES
The labial and lingual mucosa are the most frequent sites for oral warts which present as small localized growths.

DIAGNOSIS
The clinical appearance is characteristic but most lesions are removed and therefore histopathologic findings can confirm the diagnosis. Histologically, the structure is similar to papilloma but there are large clear cells (koilocytes) in the prickle cell layer. Immuno-staining may be used to detect the presence of papilloma virus.

MANAGEMENT
Excision is usually curative and recurrence is uncommon except in immunocompromised individuals.

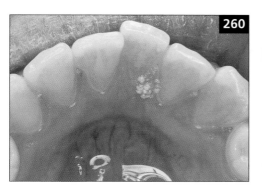

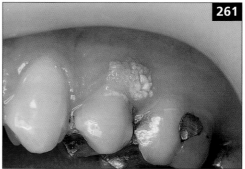

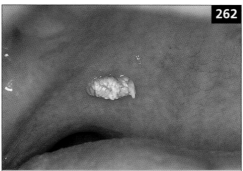

260–262 Typical 'cauliflower' appearance of squamous cell papilloma.

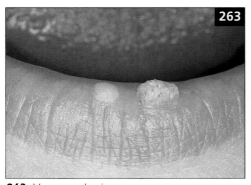

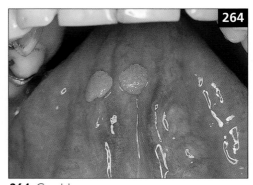

263 Verruca vulgaris.

264 Condyloma.

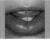

Bone exostosis

ETIOLOGY AND PATHOGENESIS
These nodular swellings consist of normal lamellar bone, although larger lesions may have a central core of cancellous bone. The cause of these exostoses is not known but an inherited autosomal dominant pattern has been described in some individuals.

CLINICAL FEATURES
Bony exostoses appear as firm swellings with normal overlying mucosa. When they occur on the midline of the hard palate they are termed torus palatinus (**265**) and when they present bilaterally on the lingual premolar region of the mandible they are termed torus mandibularis (**266, 267**). Surprisingly, torus palatinus and torus mandibularis are rarely seen together in the same individual. The prevalence of torus palatinus and torus mandibularis is 20–25% and 6–12% of the general population, respectively. Multiple bony exostoses may develop on the buccal alveolar bone of the mandible or maxilla (**268**). Frequently patients only discover a bony exostosis later in life, perhaps following a trauma which may have brought the condition to their attention, despite it having been present for several years.

DIAGNOSIS
Diagnosis is usually evident from the clinical appearance. Radiographs may be helpful to confirm the diagnosis and show dense cortical bone. Biopsy is seldom necessary.

MANAGEMENT
No active treatment is necessary, apart from reassuring the patient as to the benign nature of the condition. Since the overlying mucosa is thin and susceptible to trauma, patients may sometimes need to use an antiseptic mouthwash if ulceration develops. Occasionally a planned dental prosthesis may impinge on an exostosis, necessitating surgical removal.

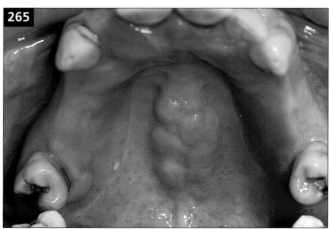

265 Torus palitinus presents as a firm, multi-nocular swelling in the middle of the palate. The overlying mucosa is normal.

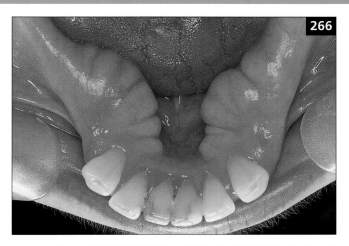

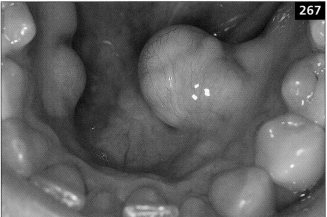

266, 267 Torus mandibularis.

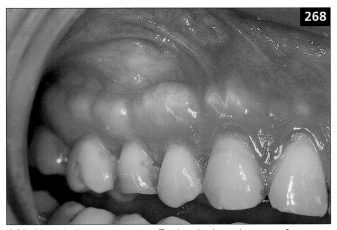

268 Multiple bone exostoses affecting the buccal aspect of the maxilla.

Sialolith (salivary stone)

ETIOLOGY AND PATHOGENESIS

A sialolith is a calcified mass or stone that can develop within the salivary glands. Such stones are believed to arise from calcium deposition around a nidus of bacteria, mucus, or ductal epithelial cells. The cause of these salivary structures is unknown, but they are not related to a systemic imbalance of calcium metabolism. A stone may develop in any major or minor salivary duct, but the submandibular gland is most frequently affected (**269**). This predilection may reflect the thick mucus secretion of the submandibular gland and the tortuous nature of its duct.

CLINICAL FEATURES

A stone will ultimately cause blockage of the salivary duct, resulting in episodic pain and rapid onset of swelling of the affected gland at meal-times. Symptoms vary and generally depend on the degree of obstruction, with larger stones more likely to produce severe and frequent symptoms. If the stone is located near the opening of the duct it may be visualized as a yellow mass that is firm to palpation (**270**).

DIAGNOSIS

Radiographs can be used to demonstrate a sialolith (**271**). About 90% of submandibular stones are radio-opaque but by contrast 90% of stones in the parotid duct are radiolucent. Stones located at the glandular end of the duct, or those that are not demonstrated by conventional radiographic imaging, may be detected using sialography.

MANAGEMENT

Small stones or those located within the duct can be manipulated towards the duct opening to allow removal. It may be necessary to incise the parotid duct orifice or the roof of the submandibular duct to gain access to the stone. In the case of large stones or those within the body of the gland, complete surgical removal of the gland may be required. In recent years, the role of lithotripsy for the disintegration and the spontaneous passage of stones is being evaluated, with some promising findings.

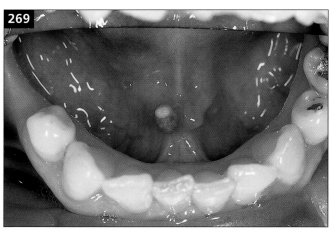

269 Salivary stone in the orifice of the submandibular duct.

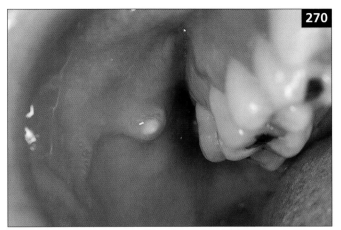

270 Salivary stone in the orifice of the parotid duct.

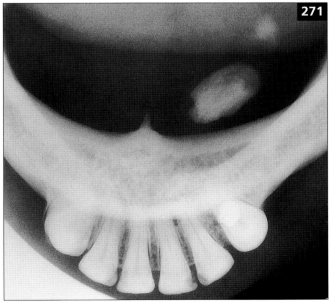

271 Radiograph showing a salivary stone in the submandibular duct.

Tongue piercing

ETIOLOGY AND PATHOGENESIS
The fashion for body art includes piercing of the orofacial tissues. Tongue piercing is particularly popular. The rich vascular and lymphatic supply of the tongue predisposes to swelling in the first few days after tongue piercing. This is also frequently complicated by secondary infection of the nonepithelialized wound.

CLINICAL FEATURES
Pronounced bilateral edema of the tongue is seen surrounding a pin or bolt at the piercing site for approximately 1 week after placement. Edema may be so pronounced that there may be risk of asphyxia. The edema will eventually resolve (**272**).

DIAGNOSIS
Diagnosis is made based on the clinical history and appearance.

MANAGEMENT
Any acute symptoms at the time of placement can be initially managed symptomatically with baking soda and water or antiseptic mouthwashes. Systemic antibiotics may be needed for cases that become secondarily infected. Emergency admission is required if the airway becomes compromised. Death has been recorded following the placement of tongue bolts.

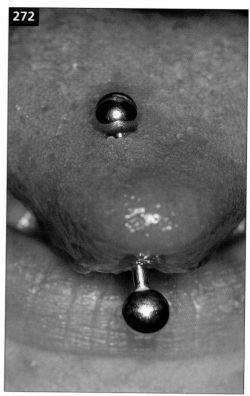

272 Tongue bolt.

Lymphoma

ETIOLOGY AND PATHOGENESIS

Lymphoma accounts for less than 5% of all oral malignancies, but can develop in any lymphoid tissue or extra-nodal site. The etiology of lymphoma is unknown, although exposure to certain toxic chemicals or high-dose radiation has been associated with the development of some forms. In addition, the Epstein–Barr virus is involved in the rare condition of Burkitt's lymphoma. Lymphoma arising in a patient with immunodeficiency, in particular infection with human immunodeficiency virus (HIV), is relatively common.

CLINICAL FEATURES

Most cases of lymphoma arise in middle-aged and elderly patients, with the exception of Burkitt's lymphoma, which is seen mostly in children and young adults. Presentation is variable and depends on the primary site and type of lymphoma. A broad division of lymphoma can be based on the site of presentation related to the lymph nodes (nodal or extra-nodal) and by histologic type (follicular or diffuse). Lymphoma arising within the lymph nodes usually presents as an asymptomatic, slowly enlarging mass. Extranodal lymphoma may also present as a mass but with pain, ulceration, or pathologic fracture. The most frequent intra-oral site is the palate (**273**). Follicular lymphomas are typically widely disseminated at presentation with bone marrow involvement. By contrast, diffuse lymphomas are usually localized to one site at presentation and patients are often spared bone marrow involvement.

DIAGNOSIS

Diagnosis is made on biopsy that shows tissue containing neoplastic lymphocytes in diffuse sheets or in a vaguely follicular pattern. Immunohistochemic and molecular analysis is required to establish definitive diagnosis and typing. Tumors are classified using the Revised European American Lymphoma (REAL) or World Health Organization (WHO) schemes, which rely on histomorphology coupled with immunophenotyping.

MANAGEMENT

Management depends on both the lymphoma type and the extent (stage) of the disease. For localized disease radiation therapy may be used, while in more widespread cases combination chemotherapy regimes are employed. The 5-year survival rate for Stage I lymphoma, treated by radiation therapy, is about 50–70%, and for Stages II–IV the figure is 30–60%. It is important to note that some lymphomas may have an indolent clinical course but are essentially incurable, while others are more rapidly dividing and yet have the best chance for cure. In general, the chance of cure is higher for a diffuse lymphoma than a follicular lymphoma.

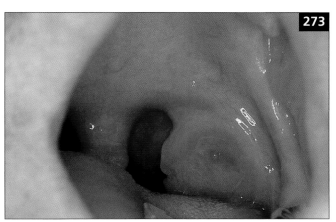

273 Lymphoma presenting as an ulcerated swelling in the soft palate. The patient was known to be HIV positive.

Pigmentation (Including Bleeding)

- **General approach**
- **Amalgam tattoo (focal agyrosis)**
- **Hemangioma (vascular nevus)**
- **Sturge–Weber syndrome**
- **Melanocytic nevus (pigmented nevus)**
- **Melanotic macule**
- **Malignant melanoma**
- **Kaposi's sarcoma**
- **Hereditary hemorrhagic telangiectasia (Rendu– Osler–Weber disease)**

- **Physiologic pigmentation**
- **Addison's disease**
- **Betel nut/pan chewing**
- **Peutz–Jegher's syndrome**
- **Black hairy tongue**
- **Drug-induced pigmentation**
- **Smoker-associated melanosis**
- **Thrombocytopenia**

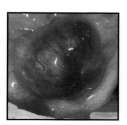
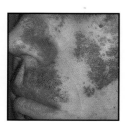
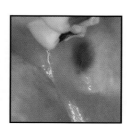
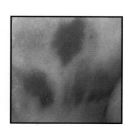

General approach

- Pigmentation of the oral mucosa may be due to melanin, blood, or foreign material.
- Pigmentation is rarely painful.
- Pigmented lesions may be either solitary or multiple.
- Pigmentation may represent neoplasia and therefore biopsy should be undertaken if there is any suspicion of malignancy or there is uncertainty of diagnosis.

Pigmentary changes can be divided on the basis of the extent of their involvement, either localized or widespread (*Table 7*).

Table 7 Pattern of pigmentation

Single or localized area of pigmentation
- Amalgam tattoo
- Hemangioma
- Melanocytic nevus (pigmented nevus)
- Melanotic macule (freckle)
- Malignant melanoma
- Kaposi's sarcoma

Multiple or widespread areas of pigmentation
- Hereditary hemorrhagic telangiectasia
- Sturge–Weber syndrome
- Physiologic pigmentation
- Addison's disease
- Betel nut/pan chewing
- Peutz–Jegher's syndrome
- Thrombocytopenia
- Black hairy tongue
- Drug-induced pigmentation
- Smoker-associated melanosis

Amalgam tattoo (focal agyrosis)

ETIOLOGY AND PATHOGENESIS

Amalgam tattoo is an iatrogenic lesion caused by the traumatic implantation of amalgam particles into the soft tissues. Such a tattoo may occur during a tooth extraction, placement of an amalgam restoration, or amalgam polishing.

CLINICAL FEATURES

Amalgam tattoo is the most frequent cause of intra-oral pigmentation and is seen on the gingivae (274), palate, buccal mucosa (275), and tongue. The tattoo appears as a slate-grey/black macule that does not change in appearance with time.

DIAGNOSIS

If there is any doubt about the clinical diagnosis, then biopsy is indicated. Histologic examination will show black particulate foreign material in the connective tissue that stains collagen fibers. If the amalgam particles are sufficiently large, they can be detected on an intra-oral radiograph.

MANAGEMENT

No treatment is required apart from establishing the diagnosis.

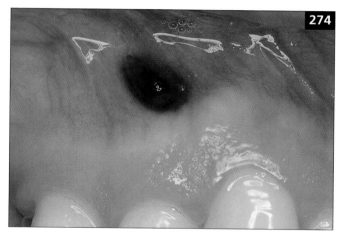

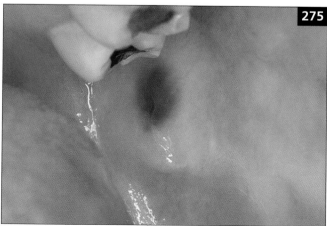

274, 275 Amalgam tattoo.

Hemangioma (vascular nevus)

ETIOLOGY AND PATHOGENESIS

Hemangioma or vascular nevus is a congenital malformation of blood vessels. The term is more often and correctly applied to the cutaneous vascular lesions of the skin that appear in infants but subsequently regress during childhood. Most oral vascular malformations are not congenital since they develop in adulthood and do not regress. However, an oral hemangioma is identical both clinically and histologically to cutaneous hemangioma. Although not strictly correct, the term hemangioma is also applied to these oral lesions. A more accurate term is probably 'vascular anomaly' or 'vascular malformation' but these names are not widely used. Hemangioma may be divided into two forms depending on the type and size of the blood vessels involved. A capillary hemangioma consists of a mass of small, fine capillary vessels whereas a cavernous hemangioma contains large, thin-wall vascular spaces.

CLINICAL FEATURES

Hemangioma may occur at any intra-oral site, although the tongue, lips, and buccal mucosa are most frequently affected. Hemangioma appear as well-circumscribed, flat or raised lesions with a blue discoloration (**276–278**).

DIAGNOSIS

Blanching of the lesion when pressure is applied to it using a glass slide (diascopy) can help confirm the diagnosis of the presence of a cavernous hemangioma (**279, 280**). Since the blood vessels of a capillary hemangioma are small, this test is not so useful for this lesion.

MANAGEMENT

The majority of cases of hemangioma do not require active treatment. However, prominent or nodular regions can become progressively traumatized and give rise to hemorrhage. If symptoms persist, small, localized lesions can be surgically excised or treated with cryotherapy. More extensive or deep lesions require specialist management including surgery and the possible use of sclerosing agents or embolization.

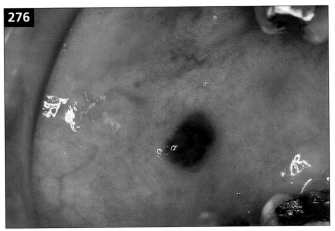

276 Hemangioma.

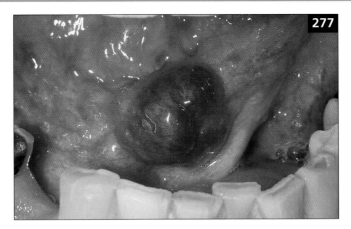

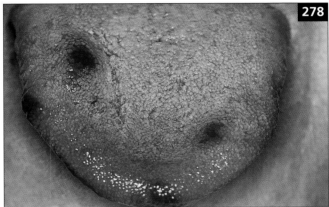

277, 278 Hemangioma.

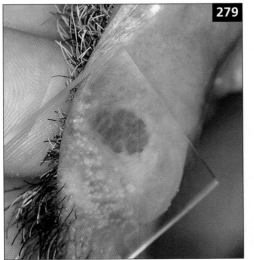

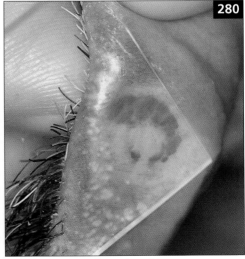

279, 280 Blanching of hemangioma following application of pressure under a glass slide.

Sturge–Weber syndrome

ETIOLOGY AND PATHOGENESIS

This congenital condition, also known as encephalotrigeminal angiomatosis, involves an angiomatous defect associated with the distribution of one or more branches of the trigeminal nerve.

CLINICAL FEATURES

The striking visible feature is the 'port wine stain' appearance of the skin of the face, which is present from birth. The capillary defect is characteristically unilateral and limited to the distribution of one branch of the trigeminal nerve. Other features include an ipsilateral leptomeningeal vascular anomaly, contralateral hemiplegia, and epilepsy. Intra-orally, the gingivae and soft tissues in the affected region may be erythematous and swollen.

DIAGNOSIS

Diagnosis is made on the clinical appearance. Plain radiographs, MRI, or CT scanning may reveal intracranial calcifications and the extent of the angiomas.

MANAGEMENT

Some patients benefit from cosmetic advice to cover facial lesions. Any dental treatment involving the extraction of teeth should be done in a hospital setting due to the risk of prolonged bleeding.

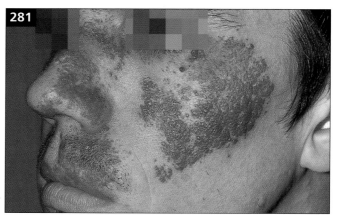

281 Characteristic facial appearance of Sturge–Weber syndrome in the maxillary division of the left trigeminal nerve.

Melanocytic nevus (pigmented nevus)

ETIOLOGY AND PATHOGENESIS

The term nevus, in a generic sense, means any congenital malformation. Unqualified or used in reference to melanocytes, the term refers to a benign neoplasm of melanocytes that is acquired or congenital. Melanocytic nevi can be junctional, compound, or intra-mucosal. Junctional nevi contain melanocytes located entirely within the epithelium, compound nevi contain melanocytes in the epithelium and in the superficial connective tissues and intra-mucosal nevi contain melanocytes only in the connective tissues. A fourth type of nevus, termed blue nevus, is composed of pigmented spindle cells located in the connective tissues. Junctional nevi mature to intra-mucosal nevi through the compound stage. Therefore, junctional nevi are most common in children, while intra-mucosal nevi are usually seen in adults. On the skin, the risk of malignant transformation of melanocytic nevi to melanoma is not entirely established. Some studies have found that one-third of melanoma contain a pre-existing melanocytic nevus. However, it is accepted that in some situations melanocytic nevus has a higher risk of malignant transformation, such as in individuals with many atypical nevi and a family history of melanoma. It has not been established if acquired melanocytic nevus of the mouth is necessarily the precursor lesion for oral melanoma. Atypical nevi have not been reported to occur in the mouth.

CLINICAL FEATURES

All oral melanocytic nevi appear as brown or blue lesions, depending on the type and depth of the melanin. The lesions have a uniform coloration, a sharply-defined border and are most often less than 0.5 cm in diameter (**282, 283**). Both junctional nevi and intra-mucosal nevi are flat but compound nevi are raised. Variations in color, indistinct borders, ulceration, and larger size are features that should prompt the consideration of malignant melanoma.

DIAGNOSIS

Diagnosis can only be made from the histological appearance of biopsy material.

MANAGEMENT

Since it is often impossible to differentiate acquired nevi from other pigmented lesions, including melanoma, all nevi should be biopsied to establish the diagnosis. Most lesions are small and therefore amenable to excisional biopsy. Once the diagnosis is established, clinical follow-up involving photographic records should be undertaken since it is still unclear if lesions may undergo malignant transformation.

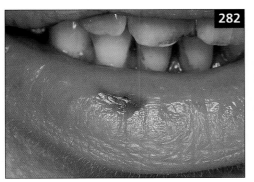
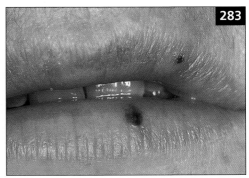

282, 283 Melanocytic nevus.

Melanotic macule

ETIOLOGY AND PATHOGENESIS
Melanotic macule is a focal pigmentation within the mouth caused by an accumulation of melanin in the epithelium and superficial connective tissues. The cause is unknown, but some macules represent intra-oral freckles and others are reactive processes to sun damage, inflammation, or trauma.

CLINICAL FEATURES
Melanotic macules appear as uniformly flat, brown macules with distinct borders usually less than 0.5 cm in size. The most common sites are the lips (284), buccal mucosa (285, 286), and gingivae. The lesions are asymptomatic but may cause esthetic problems.

DIAGNOSIS
Although the clinical features are relatively characteristic biopsy should be undertaken to obtain a definitive diagnosis.

MANAGEMENT
No treatment is required. Most macules are small and excised at time of diagnostic biopsy. In the case of multiple lesions it is helpful to take a photographic record to determine if any change in appearance occurs. A change in appearance would prompt the need for further biopsy.

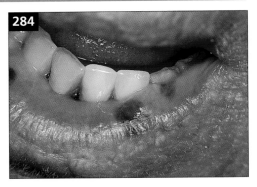

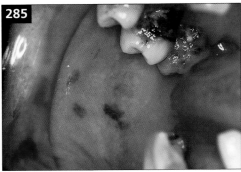

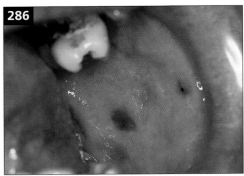

284–286 Melanotic macules.

Malignant melanoma

ETIOLOGY AND PATHOGENESIS

In contrast to malignant melanoma of the skin, where excessive exposure to ultraviolet radiation from the sun is an established risk factor, there are no known predisposing factors for intra-oral melanoma.

CLINICAL FEATURES

An intra-oral malignant melanoma may develop in clinically normal mucosa or within a pre-existing area of pigmentation. Almost all cases of melanoma contain some degree of pigmentation (**287**). Lesions can be flat or nodular, depending on the growth phase of the tumor. Clinical features that suggest melanoma include a variation in color from black to red, size less than 1 cm, irregular and poorly-defined borders, and ulceration.

DIAGNOSIS

Histolopathologic examination of biopsy material is essential for diagnosis.

MANAGEMENT

Treatment is based on radical resection of the area of involvement combined with regional lymph node dissection. Chemotherapy is often used, supplemented with immune therapy. The prognosis is based on the histologic type of melanoma and the depth of tumor invasion into the surrounding tissues. It is accepted that tumors showing deeper invasion into the connective tissues have a worse prognosis. In contrast to cutaneous melanoma, where the 5-year survival rate is about 65%, the prognosis for oral melanoma is poor, with a 5-year survival rate of around 20%. Possible factors related to the poor prognosis of oral melanoma compared to cutaneous disease include late detection, complexity of surgical excision, and an inherently more aggressive disease. In addition, oral melanoma is often accompanied by lymph node, lung, and liver involvement by the time of detection.

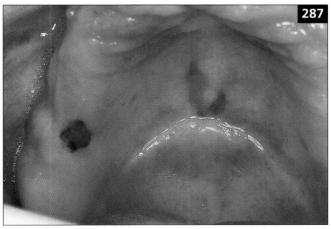

287 Malignant melanoma seen as a darkly pigmented lesion on the right palatal ridge. Note that this patient also has other areas of pigmentation.

Kaposi's sarcoma

ETIOLOGY AND PATHOGENESIS

Kaposi's sarcoma is a proliferation of endothelial cells producing a mass. A number of factors have been proposed in the development of this condition, including genetic predisposition, environmental factors, infection, and immune dysregulation. The human herpesvirus type 8 (HHV 8), also known as the Kaposi's sarcoma herpes virus (KSHV), has been identified in all forms of Kaposi's sarcoma and is now believed to be the etiologic agent.

CLINICAL FEATURES

There are three clinical forms of Kaposi's sarcoma. The classical type of lesion, first described by Kaposi in 1872, consists of red cutaneous nodules occurring on the lower extremities of older males from the Mediterranean basin. The condition has a relatively indolent course. The endemic type of Kaposi's sarcoma is seen in children and adults within Africa. The immunodeficiency type of Kaposi's is seen in adults, mostly in association with HIV infection and AIDS, but occasionally in other immunosuppressed patients. Only the immunodeficiency form is associated with oral lesions. About one-half of AIDS patients who develop Kaposi's sarcoma of the skin or viscera will develop oral lesions. The oral sites most frequently involved are the palate (**288, 289**), gingivae, and tongue. Oral Kaposi's sarcoma may present as a single lesion or at multiple sites. The clinical appearance ranges from small macules to large, nodular, exophytic masses that are red to blue in color.

DIAGNOSIS

Diagnosis is made by biopsy. Microscopically, early lesions may resemble a hemangioma or pyogenic granuloma and late lesions consist of a mass of spindle cells.

MANAGEMENT

Lesions that do not cause any functional or cosmetic problem do not require any active treatment. Small lesions can be excised, treated with low-dose radiotherapy or by the injection of a chemotherapeutic drug, such as vinblastine. Larger lesions may require the use of systemic chemotherapy.

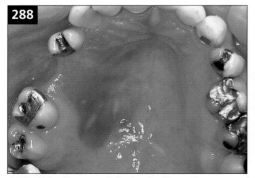
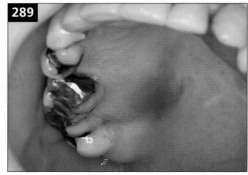

288, 289 Characteristic site for Kaposi's sarcoma in the hard palate.

Hereditary hemorrhagic telangiectasia (Rendu–Osler–Weber disease)

ETIOLOGY AND PATHOGENESIS

This rare condition is inherited in an autosomal dominant pattern. The clinical appearance is caused by the dilatation of the terminal blood vessels of the skin and mucous membranes.

CLINICAL FEATURES

Numerous telangiectatic areas appear on the skin and oral mucosa (**290**) in early life and persist throughout adulthood. Bleeding from oral lesions is a frequent problem. Intra-nasal lesions also often lead to epistaxis, which is a frequent presenting feature of this disease. If prolonged and recurrent, such bleeding can lead to anemia.

DIAGNOSIS

Diagnosis is made based on the clinical findings, particularly recurrent bleeding and a familial history of similar lesions.

MANAGEMENT

Treatment will depend on the extent of symptoms. Management of acute episodes of bleeding requires the use of surgery, cautery, or cryotherapy.

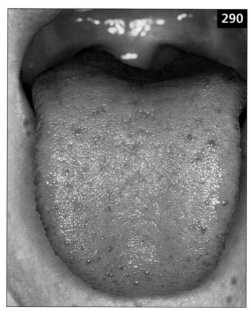

290 Multiple telangiectasia.

Physiologic pigmentation

ETIOLOGY AND PATHOGENESIS

Variations in the degree of pigmentation of the oral soft tissues are seen relatively frequently. Increased melanin production and deposition is often a physiologic process, especially in dark-skinned individuals.

CLINICAL FEATURES

Although any area of the oral mucosa may be affected, the gingivae are the most frequent site. The pigmentation can vary from brown to black and may be symmetrical or asymmetrical (**291–293**).

DIAGNOSIS

Diagnosis can be made from the clinical presentation and history but biopsy to exclude malignancy may be required if the patient reports any change in appearance.

MANAGEMENT

No treatment is required.

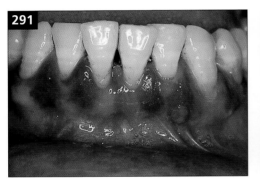

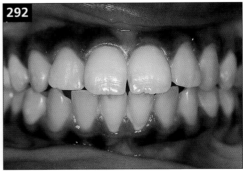

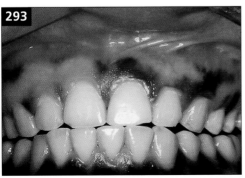

291–293 Varying degrees of physiologic pigmentation on the attached gingivae.

Addison's disease

ETIOLOGY AND PATHOGENESIS

Addison's disease is caused by a primary adreno-cortical insufficiency due to auto-immune disease, infection (usually tuberculosis), or idiopathic factors. Reduced serum levels of cortisol induces an increased production of adrenocorticotropic hormone (ACTH) resulting in hyperpigmentation of the skin and mucosal surfaces.

CLINICAL FEATURES

There is sallow hyperpigmentation of the skin similar to a sun-tan. Intra-orally, multiple melanotic macules develop on the gingivae, buccal mucosa, and lips (294). Symptoms of adrenocortical insufficiency include weakness, weight-loss, nausea and vomiting, and hypotension.

DIAGNOSIS

Biopsy of a pigmented area shows nonspecific features. Diagnosis is based on demonstrating low serum cortisol levels and elevated ACTH. Other nonspecific serum changes include low sodium, chloride, bicarbonate, and glucose.

MANAGEMENT

The condition is managed with replacement steroids. No specific treatment is required for the oral pigmentation.

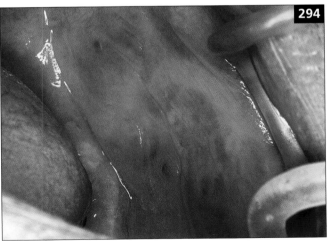

294 Pigmentation in the buccal mucosa due to Addison's disease.

Betel nut/pan chewing

ETIOLOGY AND PATHOGENESIS

Pigment in areca nut (betel) and pan may be deposited on the oral tissues.

CLINICAL FEATURES

The most striking intra-oral feature is black extrinsic staining of the teeth (**295**). However, there may also be widespread brown pigmentation of the oral mucosa, particularly the buccal mucosa and tongue (**296–298**).

DIAGNOSIS

Clinical history that reveals frequent and regular use of betel or pan.

MANAGEMENT

No treatment is required, although patients should be discouraged from the chewing of these substances due to an association with the development of submucous fibrosis (Chapter 4, p. 80) and oral squamous cell carcinoma.

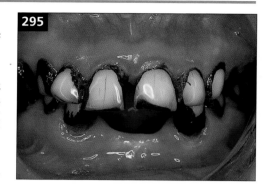

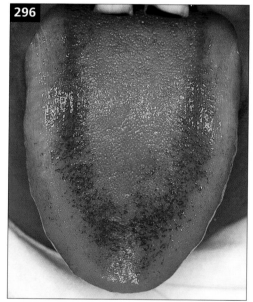

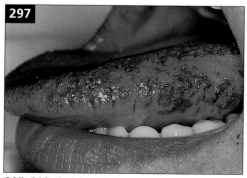

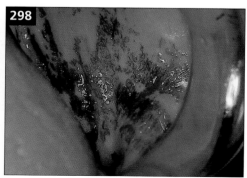

295–298 Staining of the teeth and soft tissues due to betel chewing.

Peutz–Jegher's syndrome

ETIOLOGY AND PATHOGENESIS

Peutz–Jegher's syndrome is inherited in an autosomal dominant manner and is characterized by a large number of peri-oral freckles (ephelides) and hamartomatous intestinal polyps. The condition is caused by a mutation in the *LKB1* gene which codes for a serine-threonine kinase that is thought to play a role in apoptosis.

CLINICAL FEATURES

Multiple freckles are present at the vermillion border of the lips and on the peri-oral skin (**299, 300**). Small hamartomatous polyps are present in the jejunum, colon, and gastric mucosa and are present in 75% of patients over the age of 40 years. Patients may complain of abdominal pain, rectal bleeding, and diarrhea.

DIAGNOSIS

Diagnosis is made by the clinical appearance of peri-oral freckling and a familial history of similar lesions. Biopsy of the freckles shows nonspecific features. Flexible endoscopy and biopsy may be necessary to examine the lower gastrointestinal tract for polyposis and to confirm the diagnosis.

MANAGEMENT

There is no specific treatment for the peri-oral freckles. Sunscreens may be helpful since the lesions often darken and become more prominent with sun exposure.

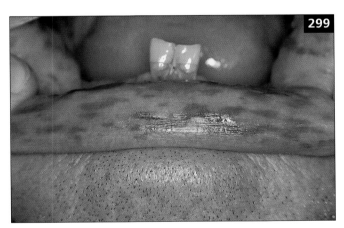

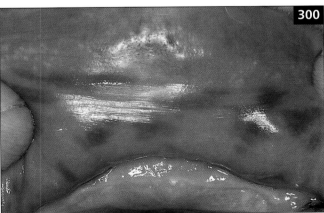

299, 300 Multiple melanotic macules in a patient with Peutz–Jegher's syndrome.

Black hairy tongue

ETIOLOGY AND PATHOGENESIS

Elongation of the filiform papillae produces a hair-like appearance on the dorsum of the tongue. The cause of the subsequent black pigmentation is unknown, although chromogenic bacteria and *Aspergillus* species have been implicated. A range of predisposing factors have been suggested, including smoking, antibiotic use, steroid therapy, and iron treatment.

CLINICAL FEATURES

The dorsum of the tongue is covered with matted, elongated, and thickened filiform papillae (**301**, **302**). The color varies from brown to dark brown. Apart from esthetic problems, there are no symptoms.

DIAGNOSIS

The clinical characteristics are so distinct that biopsy is unnecessary.

MANAGEMENT

It is important to seek the cause of black hairy tongue and, if one can be identified, then it should be eliminated. The surface of the tongue can be cleaned by vigorously brushing and by the use of a baking soda/water mouthwash. Alternatively, a tongue scraper may be useful to remove the surface layers. The patient should be reassured that the condition, although unsightly, is entirely benign.

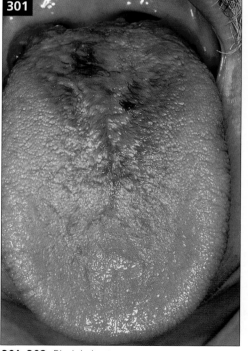

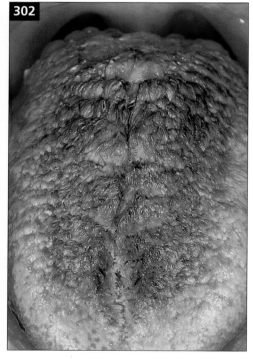

301, 302 Black hairy tongue.

Drug-induced pigmentation

ETIOLOGY AND PATHOGENESIS
A number of drugs, including minocycline, chloroquine, cyclophosphamide, azidothymidine (AZT), and amiodarone are known to have the adverse effect of intra-oral pigmentation. The mechanism is believed to be due to the stimulation of melanin production by melanocytes.

CLINICAL FEATURES
The most common intra-oral sites are the palate, buccal mucosa, and gingivae. Minocycline and chloroquine produce a characteristic bluish coloration in the midline of the hard palate (**303**). The skin can also become pigmented, particularly on sun-exposed surfaces, such as the arms and legs.

DIAGNOSIS
Diagnosis is made on the history of pigmentation following the onset of drug usage and by the clinical appearance. Biopsy may be necessary to rule out other pigmented lesions, such as melanoma, although the histology of drug-induced pigmentation is nonspecific.

MANAGEMENT
There is no specific treatment for the condition apart from discontinuation of the medication. With time there may be resolution of the pigmentation, although some lesions may persist.

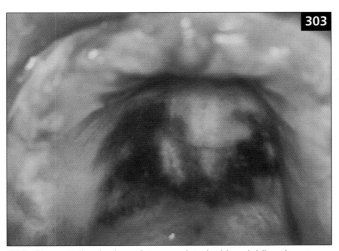

303 Pigmentation in the palate associated with quinidine therapy.

Smoker-associated melanosis

ETIOLOGY AND PATHOGENESIS
Contents of tobacco smoke are believed to stimulate melanin production by melanocytes. Hormonal factors are also likely to play a role since the condition is more common in females and in those using an oral contraceptive.

CLINICAL FEATURES
The presentation consists of diffuse pigmentation which most frequently affects the anterior labial gingivae, palate (**304**), and buccal mucosa (**305, 306**). The intensity of the pigmentation is dependent on the dose and duration of tobacco use. The condition is not seen in association with the use of smokeless tobacco products.

DIAGNOSIS
Diagnosis is made based on the clinical appearance and history of tobacco use. Biopsy shows no specific features and appears identical to physiologic pigmentation, with an increase in the amount of melanin in melanocytes and adjacent keratinocytes.

MANAGEMENT
There is no specific treatment for the condition, apart from encouraging cessation of smoking. The pigmentation usually resolves with time if the tobacco habit is eliminated.

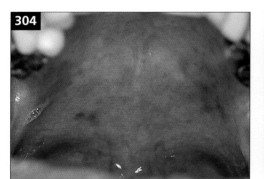

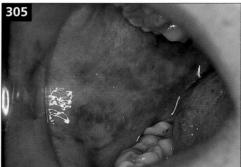

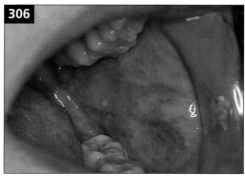

304–306 Mucosal pigmentation secondary to a smoking habit.

Thrombocytopenia

ETIOLOGY AND PATHOGENESIS

Thrombocytopenia is defined as a reduction in the number of circulating platelets below normal. There are three main causes of thrombocytopenia: an inadequate production of platelets by the bone marrow; an increased destruction in peripheral tissues; or splenic sequestration. Clinical settings in which thrombocytopenia may occur include bone marrow failure (aplastic anemia), leukemia, cancer metastasis in the bone marrow, AIDS, drug reactions, hypersplenism, post-tranfusion, immune complex formation, and the production of anti-platelet IgG antibodies.

CLINICAL FEATURES

Petechiae and pupura are seen on the skin and mucosa (**307**, **308**). There is easy bruising and spontaneous gingival bleeding (**309**). Epistaxis, melena, hematuria, and increased menstrual bleeding are also common signs.

DIAGNOSIS

Diagnosis is made hematologically on a blood count showing platelet numbers below $150 \times 10^9/l$. Microscopic examination of the blood and bone marrow will also be necessary in an attempt to determine the underlying cause of thrombocytopenia.

MANAGEMENT

Treatment is directed at the identification and correction of the cause of thrombocytopenia. For idiopathic thrombocytopenia (ITP) steroids are the treatment of choice, often with splenectomy.

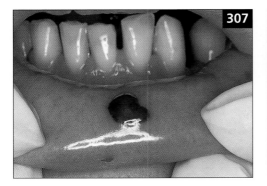
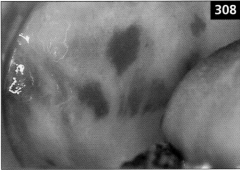
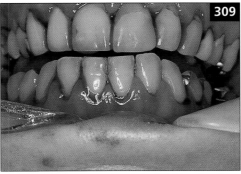

307–309 Sub-mucosal and gingival bleeding due to thrombocytopenia.

Orofacial Pain (Including Sensory and Motor Disturbance)

- **General approach**
- **Trigeminal neuralgia**
- **Glossopharyngeal neuralgia**
- **Post-herpetic neuralgia**
- **Giant cell arteritis**
- **Burning mouth syndrome**
- **Atypical facial pain**
- **Atypical odontalgia**
- **Temporomandibular joint dysfunction (TMJ dysfunction)**
- **Facial nerve palsy (Bell's palsy)**
- **Trigeminal nerve paresthesia or anesthesia**

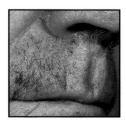
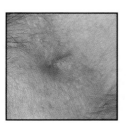
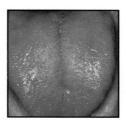
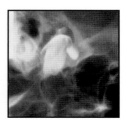

General approach

- Orofacial pain is often the reason why a patient attends a dental clinic. In most cases, clinical examination will reveal an obvious dental cause of the symptoms, such as a carious tooth, lost restoration, or acute dento-alveolar abscess. In such circumstances, diagnosis is usually relatively straightforward and appropriate treatment can be provided. (Pain of dental origin is not covered in this book.)
- Patients may also present with pain for which there is no apparent dental cause, either clinically or radiographically. In this case a diagnosis can only be made on the basis of a detailed assessment of the character of the pain, including factors such as duration, site, severity, initiating factors, and relieving factors. Clinical examination and questioning will reveal other typical findings associated with each condition.

Orofacial pain can be initially divided into those conditions in which symptoms are episodic and those in which the pain is constant (*Tables 8–10*). This chapter also covers neurologic disorders that may present as either altered sensation or loss of motor function.

Table 8 Pattern of pain

Episodic pain
- Trigeminal neuralgia
- Glossopharyngeal neuralgia
- Post-herpetic neuralgia
- Giant cell arteritis

Constant pain
- Burning mouth syndrome
- Atypical facial pain
- Atypical odontalgia
- Post-herpetic neuralgia
- Temporomandibular joint dysfunction

Loss of function or sensation
- Facial nerve palsy
- Trigeminal nerve paresthesia

Table 9 Episodic pain symptoms

	Trigeminal neuralgia	Glossopharyngeal neuralgia	Giant cell arteritis
Site	Face	Throat, tonsillar region	Temple
Nature	Sharp, stabbing, shooting	Sharp, stabbing, shooting	Dull ache
Severity	Worst pain experienced	Worst pain experienced	Severe
Initiating factors	Light touch, washing	Swallowing, chewing	Eating
Relieving factors	None	None	None

Table 10 Constant pain symptoms

	Burning mouth syndrome	Atypical facial pain	Atypical odontalgia
Site	Mouth	Face	Tooth
Nature	Burning	Dull, boring ache	Dull, boring toothache
Severity	Moderate to severe	Moderate to severe	Moderate to severe
Initiating factors	None	None	None
Relieving factors	None	None	None

Trigeminal neuralgia

ETIOLOGY AND PATHOGENESIS

A number of theories have been proposed as to the etiology of trigeminal neuralgia. Histopathologic examination of autopsy material from patients with a history of trigeminal neuralgia has led to a suggestion that pain occurs due to the presence of areas of demyelination along the distribution of the trigeminal nerve, particularly where the nerve exits the base of the skull. Alternatively, other studies using MRI have implicated the involvement of aberrant intracranial blood vessels in the cerebello-pontine region. Rarely, an accompanying organic disease such as a neoplasm within the nasopharynx, maxillary antrum, middle ear, or base of the skull, or a vascular aneurysm in close relation to the trigeminal nerve may produce symptoms attributable to trigeminal neuralgia. Trigeminal neuralgia is a relatively common condition in older individuals; however, diagnosis in a patient under the age of 40 years should raise suspicion of the presence of an underlying systemic disease, in particular multiple sclerosis or HIV infection.

CLINICAL FEATURES

The pain of trigeminal neuralgia is characteristic in that it is unilateral and limited to the anatomic pathway of one of the three main branches (mandibular, maxillary, or ophthalmic) of the trigeminal nerve. The pain is of short duration, lasting only a matter of seconds. However, despite being brief, the severity of the symptoms is extreme and many patients report that the pain is the worst that they have ever experienced. The nature of the pain is shooting, stabbing or 'electric-shock'-like. Sufferers may describe trigger spots on their skin or in their mouth, while others report that smiling, eating, or washing can bring on an attack. In males, such a trigger spot may prevent shaving in a particular area, resulting in an area of facial hair growth (**310**). Clinical examination will not reveal any abnormality apart from the site of any trigger spots. Indeed, intra-oral examination may be complicated or limited due to the patient's fear that movement or contact with facial tissues may precipitate an attack of pain. The presence of any other neurologic signs or symptoms, such as muscle weakness or altered nerve sensation, would indicate the need for a full neurologic assessment.

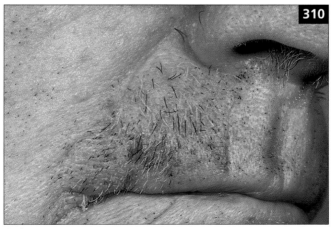

310 Unshaven area due to a trigger spot on the upper lip.

DIAGNOSIS

Diagnosis is based on the clinical history and the nature of the symptoms. Although not practical in many clinical settings, it has been suggested that a CT or MRI scan should be performed on any patient suspected of having trigeminal neuralgia to rule out organic disease, such as a brainstem tumor.

MANAGEMENT

Trigeminal neuralgia can usually be successfully managed pharmacologically using the anticonvulsant drug, carbamazepine. Initial treatment should comprise 100 mg carbamazepine, taken every 8 hours. It is likely that this will have to be increased over the subsequent days to achieve full control of the pain. In practice a dose of 600–800 mg, in divided dosages, is usually required. Carbamazepine may be given up to levels of 1,600 mg/day. The half-life of carbamazepine varies, depending on the frequency of the dosage prescribed, and therefore the more frequently the drug is administered the shorter the half-life. If a regimen of divided doses fails to control the pain, it is worthwhile trying a single or two-dose approach. Alternatively, therapy may be changed to a modified release preparation, carbamazepine retard.

The duration of treatment remains speculative but most patients can gradually reduce therapy after 6–12 symptom-free months. Prescribing the drug for short periods of time (1–2 months) will almost certainly result in a recurrence of pain. Carbamazepine therapy has recognized side-effects of suppression of white cell production and induction of liver enzymes. In view of these effects, baseline full blood count (FBC) and liver function tests (LFTs) should be taken prior to the start of therapy. These tests should be repeated at approximately 3-monthly intervals while treatment is being given. If a progressive neutropenia is encountered then the drug should be changed. In the first instance, a more recent preparation, oxcarbazepine (not available in the US), which may be given at levels of up to 2,400 mg per day with reduced likelihood of inducing neutropenia, may be tried. In addition, carbamazepine may produce other adverse events, in particular nausea, ataxia, and an erythematous, pruritic skin rash. Cases of erythema multiforme have also been reported in association with the use of carbamazepine.

If carbamazepine therapy is found to be ineffective or has to be discontinued because of the side-effects mentioned above, then consideration can be given to the use of phenytoin, clonazepam, sodium valproate, or gabapentin. Should all types of medical therapy fail then surgical treatment may have to be considered. Peripheral techniques involving alcohol or glycerol nerve blocks are effective in some cases, although symptoms do return after approximately 18 months. Cryotherapy, surgical section, fractional rhizotomy, or thermocoagulation have also been tried, with varying success. Unfortunately, surgical techniques produce permanent facial anesthesia and a risk of dysesthia, which can be troublesome to the patient. Microvascular decompression (MVD) is a neurosurgical procedure involving displacement of aberrant blood vessels from immediate contact with the trigeminal nerve. MVD has achieved a high success rate but the use of this technique should be considered on an individual basis due to the significant risks of morbidity or mortality.

Glossopharyngeal neuralgia

ETIOLOGY AND PATHOGENESIS

The etiology of glossophayngeal neuralgia is uncertain. However, since the symptoms of this condition are like those of trigeminal neuralgia, similar mechanisms may be involved. In contrast, glossopharyngeal neuralgia is a rare condition and tends to affect a slightly younger age group than trigeminal neuralgia. It is important to remember that cases of glossopharyngeal neuralgia are often found to represent the presence of a neoplasm at the base of the tongue or in the oropharynx.

CLINICAL FEATURES

The pain of glossopharyngeal neuralgia is identical to trigeminal neuralgia (above), but in this condition the severe shooting sensation is sited within the tonsil region or oropharynx, possibly with radiation to the ear. The symptoms are usually initiated by swallowing, chewing, or coughing.

DIAGNOSIS

Diagnosis is based on the clinical history and the nature of the symptoms. As with trigeminal neuralgia, the presence of organic disease, in particular pharyngeal carcinoma or salivary gland neoplasm, should be excluded by appropriate examination of the oropharynx supplemented with a CT scan (**311**) or MRI.

MANAGEMENT

Carbamazepine is usually successful in controlling the pain. Resolution of symptoms following a trial course of carbamazepine in a suspected case can support the diagnosis. Surgical options may be considered in cases that are unresponsive to drug therapy.

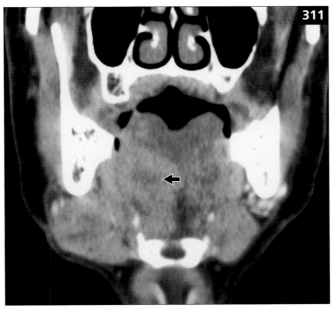

311 CT scan showing squamous cell carcinoma at the base of the tongue (arrow).

Post-herpetic neuralgia

ETIOLOGY AND PATHOGENESIS
Approximately 10% of patients who have suffered recurrent varicella zoster infection of the trigeminal nerve (shingles, herpes zoster) subsequently develop persistent neuralgia. Damage to neural tissue or the persistence of varicella zoster virus within the trigeminal nerve have been implicated in this condition.

CLINICAL FEATURES
The pain is varied in character, ranging from episodic, severe, shooting pain to a constant burning sensation. The affected area may show signs of post-inflammatory pigmentation or scarring from the preceding episode of herpes zoster (312–314).

DIAGNOSIS
Diagnosis is made on the nature of the symptoms and the previous history of shingles.

MANAGEMENT
Post-herpetic neuralgia is extremely resistant to treatment. Provision of carbamazepine, phenytoin, or gabapentin is rarely effective. Similarly surgical approaches produce no benefit. Transcutaneous electric nerve stimulation (TENS) has found to be of some help in certain patients.

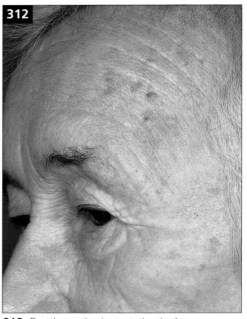

312 Post-herpetic pigmentation in the distribution of the ophthalmic nerve.

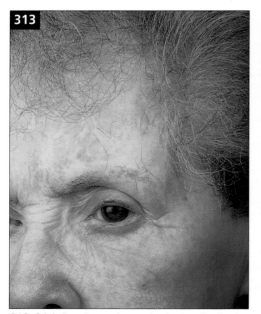

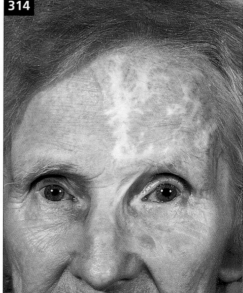

313, 314 Post-herpetic scarring in the distribution of the ophthalmic nerve.

Giant cell arteritis

ETIOLOGY AND PATHOGENESIS

Giant cell arteritis is a granulomatous vasculitis that was previously termed temporal arteritis. The latter term was replaced since the condition was found to affect vessels in the head or neck other than the temporal artery. If untreated, patients may develop retinal vasculitis with a subsequent loss of sight.

CLINICAL FEATURES

The condition generally occurs in individuals over the age of 60 years and principally presents as unilateral 'headache-like' pain in the temporal or occipital region. It is one of the few causes of orofacial pain in which patients describe systemic upset, including weight-loss, muscle weakness, and lethargy, although muscle biopsy, enzymology, and electromyography are normal. The pain can be initiated by eating and therefore the patient can only eat for short periods before resting to allow the pain to subside. This limitation of normal eating is thought to be ischemic in origin and has been misnamed 'jaw claudication'.

DIAGNOSIS

Hematologic investigation will usually show a raised erythrocyte sedimentation rate (ESR) and possibly raised c-reactive protein (CRP). It has been proposed that temporal artery biopsy (315) is of value in confirming the diagnosis; however, the granulomatous lesions occur sporadically along the vessel (skip lesions) and therefore several biopsies may be required to detect them. More importantly, the delay in obtaining the results of such a biopsy can be hazardous due to the possible onset of blindness.

MANAGEMENT

Treatment should start immediately if a diagnosis of giant cell arteritis is suspected. Oral prednisolone (prednisone) at a dose of 40–60 mg daily is a routine initial management. After symptoms have been controlled the therapy can be reduced, although a low maintenance dose may be required for 3–6 months. The ESR is a reasonable guide to disease activity and this should fall to normal levels (<20 mm/hr) following institution of steroid therapy.

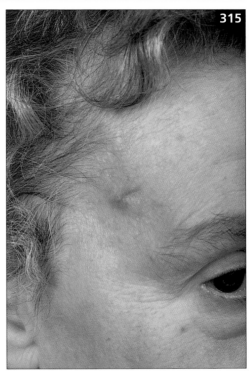

315 Scar at the site of a temporal artery biopsy.

Burning mouth syndrome

ETIOLOGY AND PATHOGENESIS

A variety of terms, such as glossopyrosis, glossodynia, stomatopyrosis, stomatodynia, and oral dysesthesia, have been used to describe a complaint of a burning sensation affecting the oral mucosa in the absence of any obvious mucosal abnormality. In recent years the term 'burning mouth syndrome' (BMS) has been used increasingly in this situation. The etiology of BMS is uncertain although a number of factors have been suggested, including hematinic deficiency (vitamin B complex, iron or folic acid), undiagnosed or poorly controlled diabetes, candidosis, denture design faults, xerostomia, and food allergy. Almost invariably patients with BMS are found to have anxiety or depression related to previous or current adverse life events.

CLINICAL FEATURES

BMS predominantly affects females but can occasionally develop in males. Generally, older individuals are affected, with a peak incidence between 50–60 years of age. The burning is invariably constant, although in some sufferers the symptoms tend to become more severe as the day progresses. The patient often has a poor sleep pattern and will report early-morning waking, a recognized indicator of depression. Any area may be affected, although the lips and the tongue are most frequently involved. Examination of the mouth in BMS will fail to reveal any mucosal abnormality (**316**). Sometimes the patient may express concern about particular areas within the mouth but these are usually found to be prominent lingual papillae (**9, 10**), minor salivary glands, or ectopic sebaceous glands (**14**).

DIAGNOSIS

Diagnosis can be made clinically on the basis of a complaint of oral burning in the absence of any mucosal abnormality. Hematologic investigations to exclude hematinic deficiency and diabetes mellitus should be undertaken. The presence of candida can be detected by taking a smear, swab, imprint culture, or oral rinse. Since tongue rubbing is often an important cause of localized burning, it is necessary to examine the teeth, dental restorations, or prostheses for possible traumatic edges. Any dentures worn by the patients should be examined for inadequate design and evidence of wear facets (**317**). Stimulated parotid flow rates should be measured if there is a clinical indication of xerostomia. The presence of a parafunctional habit may be seen as scalloped lateral margins of the tongue.

The severity of burning should be recorded on a ten-point scale where zero is 'no burning' and ten is the 'worst burning possible'. The degree of cancerphobia can be assessed by asking the patient to rate fear of oral cancer on a scale of zero to ten, where zero indicates 'no concern of cancer' and ten indicates 'an overwhelming concern of cancer'. The presence of adverse home circumstances or life events can also be detected using a similar scale, where zero corresponds to 'things could not be worse' and ten indicates that 'things could not be better'. This type of questioning often reveals factors such as marital problems, poor housing conditions, or illness in relatives. The Hospital Anxiety and Depression (HAD) Scale can be used to determine the likelihood of the patient having anxiety or depression.

MANAGEMENT

Treatment should initially involve reassurance of the common nature of BMS and the absence of any serious underlying problem, in particular oral cancer, since patients frequently have a significant level of cancerphobia. The patient should be reviewed with the results of the hematologic and microbiologic investigations and any abnormalities corrected. Sharp edges on teeth or restorations should be smoothed or a thin acrylic splint fabricated for continual or night-only wear.

Antidepressant therapy plays a major role in the management of BMS once other precipitating factors have been excluded. Some tricyclic drugs, such as dothiepin (doxepine) and amitriptiline (amitryptyline), have anxiolytic, antidepressant and muscle relaxant activity and have been found to be of great benefit for patients with BMS. Dothiepin, at a dose of 50–75 mg given before sleep, is a standard approach. However, dry mouth is a relatively frequent side-effect of the tricyclic drugs and therapy may have to be discontiued. Alternatively, a serotonin re-uptake inhibitor (SSRI), such as fluoxetine, fluvoxamine, or paroxetine, may be used. It has been suggested that SSRI preparations have fewer side-effects than tricyclic antidepressants, in particular less adverse effects on reaction time. The management of patients with BMS requires liaison between dental and medical practitioners. In some patients it may be necessary to seek combined specialist care from the oral physician, dermatologist, psychiatrist, or clinical psychologist.

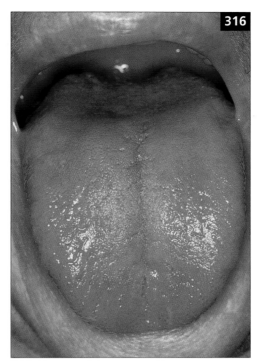

316 Dorsum of the tongue with no mucosa abnormality in burning mouth syndrome.

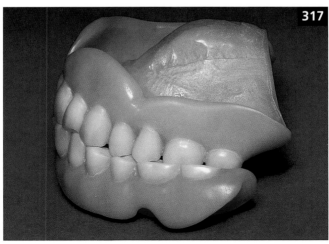

317 Full dentures with wear facets and poor occlusion.

Atypical facial pain

ETIOLOGY AND PATHOGENESIS

Atypical facial pain is a chronic pain of unknown etiology. Up to 50% of patients with atypical facial pain will be found to have anxiety or depression relating to adverse life events, although the nature of this relationship is unclear. Alternatively, there may be a prolonged history of dental disease, usually involving surgical procedures and infection, in a particular area of the mouth.

CLINICAL FEATURES

Atypical facial pain predominantly affects females over the age of 30 years. This condition is a distinct clinical entity with 'typical' symptoms consisting of a constant unilateral boring or gnawing dull ache. The pain is chronic, being present every day from the time of waking until the patient goes to sleep. These symptoms do not awaken the patient from sleep but, because the condition is often associated with depression, a sleep disturbance (in these instances early-morning waking) is often present. Although poorly localized, the pain most frequently affects one side of the maxilla. The crossing of anatomic boundaries is an occasional feature; for example, the pain may cross the midline of the maxilla or mandible. Clinical examination will fail to reveal any abnormality but radiographs of the affected region must be taken to exclude the presence of dental or maxillary antral disease (**318**).

DIAGNOSIS

Diagnosis is made on the basis of the clinical history and the absence of any dental cause of the pain. An assessment of cranial nerve function should be undertaken and a CT scan or MRI performed if any abnormality is detected to exclude malignancy at the base of the skull. The Hospital Anxiety and Depression (HAD) scale is helpful to determine the presence of anxiety or depression.

MANAGEMENT

Atypical facial pain responds well to low-dose antidepressive drug therapy. Dothiepin, 50–75 mg before sleep, is the drug regime of choice. Alternatively, amitriptiline (amitryptyline) or nortriptyline beginning at 25 mg nightly has also been used successfully. Typically a small dose is initiated and gradually escalated incrementally until the pain is controlled. In recent years, fluoxetine, fluvoxamine, paroxetine, and venlafaxine have also been used in the management of this condition. Irrespective of which drug is chosen, therapy needs to be provided for at least 6 months.

Atypical odontalgia

ETIOLOGY AND PATHOGENESIS

This condition is closely related to atypical facial pain and is likely to have a similar psychologic component. Many cases have a long and complicated history of failed dental treatment, although this relationship is poorly defined.

CLINICAL FEATURES

The complaint is of a constant dull ache, which is boring in nature. The symptoms are localized to one tooth or edentulous area that is clinically and radiographically normal.

DIAGNOSIS

Diagnosis is based on the clinical history and the absence of dental pathology. The Hospital Anxiety and Depression (HAD) scale can be used to determine the presence of anxiety or depression.

MANAGEMENT

Treatment is based on the use of antidepressant therapy, such as dothiepin 50–75 mg, amitriptiline (amitryptyline) 25–75 mg or fluoxetine 20 mg, taken before sleep.

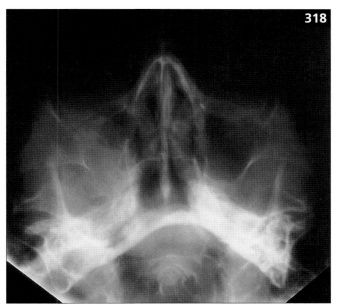

318 Occipitomental radiograph showing a radio-opaque mass in the right maxillary antrum. This lesion was found to be a carcinoma. The presenting symptoms were similar to atypical facial pain.

Temporomandibular joint dysfunction (TMJ dysfunction)

ETIOLOGY AND PATHOGENESIS

The etiology of TMJ dysfunction remains a subject of divided opinion, despite considerable research into the condition. Confusion in the literature may in part be due to the variety of terms that have been used to describe the complaint, which has included facial pain dysfunction, myofacial pain dysfunction, and facial arthromyalgia. Although the cause of TMJ dysfunction remains uncertain, it is likely to be associated with one or more of the following factors: occlusal abnormalities; lack of posterior teeth; parafunctional clenching habits; nocturnal bruxism; anxiety; and depression. Occasionally, a patient may relate the onset of pain to an acute incident of local trauma while eating or yawning.

CLINICAL FEATURES

The symptoms consist of a constant dull unilateral or bilateral pre-auricular or auricular pain that can undergo acute exacerbations, which radiate to the temple, maxilla, or occipital regions. In addition the patient may complain of trismus, limited jaw movements, tenderness of the joint, and headache. Common to all is pain on chewing, yawning, or talking. Clinical examination is likely to reveal tenderness of one or both of the temporomandibular joints and associated muscles of mastication. An audible click may be present on jaw movement. There may be evidence of bruxism in the form of wear facets on the teeth. Lack of posterior teeth combined with an absence of partial dentures is another occasional association. Radiographic examination of the joints is usually unnecessary because in the majority of cases there is no visible abnormality. However, in some cases a panoramic radiograph will show gross loss of the alveolar bone (**319**) and lack of support for satisfactory wearing of complete dentures.

DIAGNOSIS

Diagnosis is made from the clinical history and examination. It is important to differentiate between TMJ dysfunction, which involves abnormal physical activity of the joint, and TMJ diseases in which there is a pathological change of the joint. Radiographic assessment including arthrography of the temporomandibular joint may be required if the presenting signs and symptoms suggest the presence of structural TMJ disease (**320, 321**).

MANAGEMENT

Opinions on the treatment of TMJ dysfunction are widely divided. However, the provision of a hard acrylic splint with full occlusal coverage that is worn at night successfully improves the symptoms in many patients. The decision to construct either an upper or lower splint with a flat occlusal surface can be determined on the basis of the number and position of the teeth present in each arch. Rest and limitation of movement, supplemented with moist heat applied to the affected joint and muscle, can provide significant improvement in the condition. In acute or severe cases it can be helpful to provide a mild anxiolytic and muscle relaxant, such as diazepam, for a few days. Tricyclic antidepressant therapy has also been found to produce symptomatic improvement and can be considered when splint treatment is either not feasible or fails to be effective. The technique of arthrocentesis has also been reported to be useful but its value for all patients remains unclear.

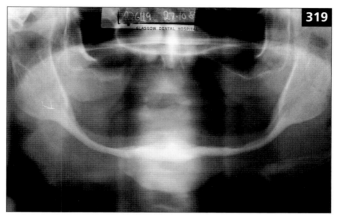

319 Orthopantomograph of an edentulous individual showing gross loss of the alveolar bone.

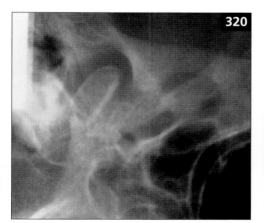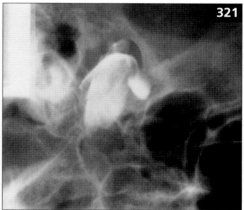

320, 321 Plain view and arthrogram of the temporomandibular joint. Radio-opaque contrast medium has been injected locally to demonstrate the architecture of the upper and lower joint spaces.

Facial nerve palsy (Bell's palsy)

ETIOLOGY AND PATHOGENESIS
Facial nerve palsy can occur either because of a stroke (upper motor lesion) or Bell's palsy (lower motor lesion). The site of the lesion is important since the muscles of the upper part of the face receive bilateral innervation, while those in the lower part of the face have a unilateral input from the contralateral motor cortex only. Bell's palsy is due to an inflammatory pressure effect on the facial nerve as it passes through the stylomastoid canal. Inflammation or fluid pressure at this site often develops in pregnancy or in viral infection involving herpes simplex or varicella zoster viruses. Tumors of the base of the skull or the parotid gland can also produce pressure on the facial nerve resulting in Bell's palsy.

CLINICAL FEATURES
Upper motor lesions present with a unilateral facial palsy, although there is some function of frontalis and orbicularis oculi. The presence of paresis in the arm or leg on the affected side would also support an upper motor defect. In the case of lower motor lesions the unilateral paralysis is total, with the absence of voluntary movements of the facial muscles.

DIAGNOSIS
The patient should be asked to perform a series of facial muscles movements, including furrowing of the forehead (**322**), raising of the eyebrows, closure of the eyes, whistling, and smiling (**323**). A tumor of the salivary gland must be ruled out by clinical examination supplemented with radiographic assessment.

MANAGEMENT
The function of the other cranial nerves, in particular V and VI, should be tested. The external ear should be examined and the hearing assessed. Bell's palsy should be treated promptly with high-dose corticosteroid therapy (40–50 mg oral prednisolone [prednisone]) and systemic antiviral therapy, such as aciclovir (acyclovir) or famciclovir. An eye-patch should be provided to limit the possibility of damage to the cornea. Most cases of Bell's palsy resolve within 3–4 weeks. The steroid therapy can be reduced gradually during this time in relation to the return of nerve function. Unfortunately, if untreated the palsy may be permanent.

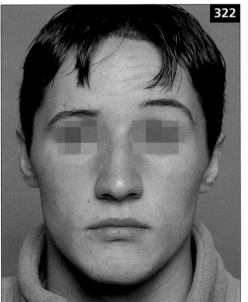

322 Facial nerve palsy preventing the furrowing of the right side of the forehead.

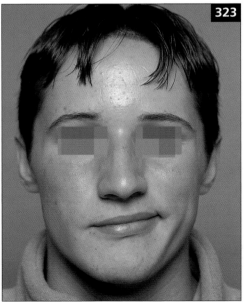

23 Facial nerve palsy preventing the elevation of the right corner of the mouth while the patient attempts to smile.

Trigeminal nerve paresthesia or anesthesia

ETIOLOGY AND PATHOGENESIS

In addition to direct trauma to the nerve, altered function can be the presenting feature of both benign and malignant neoplasms within the head and neck. Alternatively, nerve dysfunction may follow a viral infection since many viruses, in particular members of the herpes group, are neurotropic and reside in latent form within the sensory nerves. Iron deficiency and diabetes have also been implicated as a cause of altered sensory nerve function.

CLINICAL FEATURES

Patients most frequently complain of a sudden onset of a unilateral, partial, or complete loss of sensation within the distribution of one trigeminal nerve. All three branches of the nerve are usually affected. Occasionally the onset is gradual and affects only one branch of the nerve.

DIAGNOSIS

Tactile and pin-prick testing can confirm the loss of function (324). CT scanning or MRI should be used to detect the presence of any pathology associated with the trigeminal nerve (325).

MANAGEMENT

Initial management should involve the assessment of the 12 cranial nerves. Clinical examination should exclude any other extra-oral and intra-oral pathology. Hematologic tests should include the assessment of iron status and glucose.

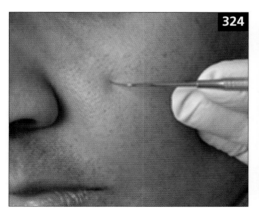

324 Pin prick test.

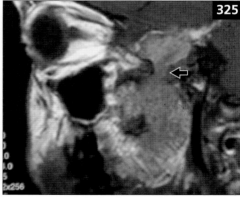

325 MRI scan showing tumor penetrating the foramen ovale (arrow) from the middle cranial fossa leading to destruction of the trigeminal nerve. The patient presented with anesthesia in the distribution of the mandibular nerve.

Dry Mouth, Excess Salivation, Coated Tongue, Halitosis, and Altered Taste

- **General approach**
- **Xerostomia (dry mouth)**
- **Sjögren's syndrome**
- **CREST syndrome**
- **Excess salivation (sialorrhea)**
- **Coated tongue**
- **Halitosis (bad breath)**
- **Altered taste**

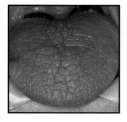
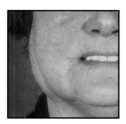
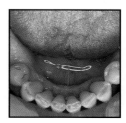
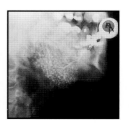

General approach

- Although the presence of xerostomia or excess salivation can usually be determined easily, the successful management of these conditions involves a range of clinical and special investigations to determine the underlying cause.

- The tongue has a natural degree of white coating in health. However, this coating can become excessive or undergo color change.
- Bad breath (halitosis) or altered taste is a frequent complaint. This usually represents an oral hygiene problem but an underlying disease should not be excluded if a local cause cannot be found.

Xerostomia (dry mouth)

ETIOLOGY AND PATHOGENESIS

A reduced production of saliva is usually due to one of the following: an effect of drug therapy; an immune-related disease; radiation damage; or dehydration. Anxiety may also limit the production of saliva, both on an acute or a chronic basis. Xerostomia due to congenital abnormalities or development failure of the salivary glands is extremely rare.

CLINICAL FEATURES

The clinical presentation of xerostomia or reduced salivary production is the same, regardless of the cause. Patients complain of a number of symptoms, in particular difficulty in talking or swallowing, altered taste, generalized oral discomfort and, if worn, poor retention of dentures. A reduction in saliva flow of less than 50% is usually required before clinical symptoms develop. Examination will reveal a lack of saliva in the floor of the mouth and attempts to express saliva from the major salivary duct openings by external pressure on the gland may fail. In addition to being reduced in amount, any saliva that is present may be frothy in nature (**326**). The buccal mucosa becomes sticky and will adhere to the face of a dental mirror placed against it. Lack of saliva will produce a generalized erythema of the oral mucosa (**327**, **328**) and a lobulated appearance on the dorsum of the tongue (**329**). There is also likely to be evidence of candidosis (candidiasis) and angular cheilitis. The teeth are prone to cervical caries and existing restorations may fail due to recurrent caries (**330**, **331**). Patients with xerostomia are also predisposed to recurrent episodes of suppurative sialadenitis, particularly of the parotid gland (Chapter 6, p. 98).

DIAGNOSIS

Xerostomia can be diagnosed clinically on the basis of little or no saliva pooling in the floor of the mouth at rest. Unfortunately, determination of the underlying cause of xerostomia may be problematic and requires a range of special investigations. The patient's medical history may reveal the possibility of drug-induced xerostomia, particularly if the onset of symptoms coincided with the provision of a new medication. Drugs that are known to produce xerostomia include: antidepressants; antihistamines; anti-cholinergic agents; potent diuretics; and narcotics. Similarly, a history of previous radiotherapy to the head and neck region, renal failure, or hemorrhage will be gained from the patient. Hematologic investigation should include fasting blood glucose, urea and electrolytes. Additional hematologic tests and other special investigations, including sialography and scintiscanning, are required if Sjögren's syndrome is suspected (*Table 11* and p. 18).

MANAGEMENT

If xerostomia is due to an adverse drug reaction then consideration should be given to changing the patient's medication, although this may not always be possible, particularly when there is a long history of antidepressant therapy. Xerostomia due to undiagnosed or poorly-controlled diabetes should improve once glycemic control is achieved. In the case of immune-related disease or post-radiotherapy damage, little can be done to correct the deficiency and management is limited to minimizing the effects of lack of saliva.

Artificial saliva substitutes, based on either carboxymethylcellulose or mucin, are commercially available and provide a source of saliva replacement. However, the use of such preparations is unsatisfactory since, although a degree of relief is gained, this lasts for a few minutes only. Artificial saliva is relatively expensive and has little advantage over water. Chewing of sugar-free gum or pastilles produces salivary flow from the remaining functional tissue and is found to be helpful by many patients. Salivary stimulants (sialogues) based on glycerine and lemon preparations should only be used in edentulous patients since their low pH will encourage dental caries in dentate individuals. The role of systemic pilocarpine, a stimulant of exocrine glands secretion, has been disappointing since, although salivary flow can be obtained prior to meals, patients often complain of significant adverse events, in particular sweating. Rigorous oral hygiene measures and preventive regimens, such as daily fluoride mouthwash or professionally applied topical fluoride therapy, should be instituted to reduce the risk of dental caries. Dietary advice should be given, especially concerning the limitation of sugar intake.

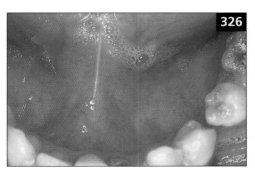

326 'Frothy' saliva.

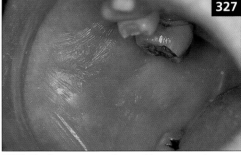

327 Erythematous and atrophic mucosa due to xerostomia.

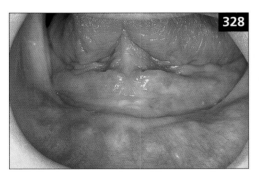

328 Erythematous and atrophic mucosa due to xerostomia.

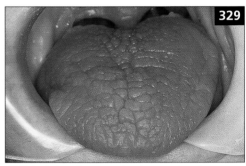

329 Lobulated tongue due to xerostomia.

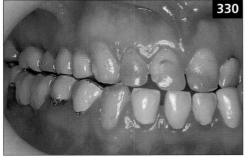

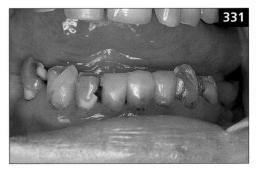

330, 331 Failing restorations in xerostomia.

Sjögren's syndrome

ETIOLOGY AND PATHOGENESIS

Henrick Sjögren first described an association between dry mouth and dry eyes in 1933. Since then further work has revealed an involvement of connective tissue disorders and auto-immune disease. Two forms of Sjögren's syndrome are now recognized. Primary Sjögren's syndrome, previously referred to as sicca syndrome, consists of dry eyes and dry mouth. In secondary Sjögren's syndrome, the patient has a connective tissue disorder in addition to suffering from dry eyes and/or dry mouth. Sjögren's syndrome is a relatively common condition and it has been estimated that approximately 15% of patients with rheumatoid arthritis are affected.

CLINICAL FEATURES

Patients with secondary Sjögren's syndrome are likely to show obvious extra-oral manifestations of rheumatoid arthritis (**332**), systemic lupus erythematosus (**333**), progressive systemic sclerosis, or primary biliary cirrhosis. In the case of primary Sjögren's syndrome, the signs and symptoms are limited to the mouth and the eyes. The oral manifestations are as described above for any cause of dry mouth. Swelling of the parotid salivary glands occurs in approximately one-third of cases of Sjögren's syndrome (**334**).

DIAGNOSIS

Diagnosis of Sjögren's syndrome, using the European classification criteria, is based on the compilation of the results of a range of clinical observations and special investigations, including measurement of salivary flow rates, assessment of lacrimal flow (Schirmer's test) (**35**), labial gland biopsy (**34**), sialography (**335**), and immunological studies for markers in venous blood (*Table 11*).

MANAGEMENT

The treatment of the oral component of Sjögren's syndrome is identical to that for any cause of dry mouth (pp. 166–167). Salivary lymphoepithelial lesions, also known as benign lymphoepithelial lesions or myoepithelial sialadenitis, are seen in Sjögren's syndrome and may progress to B-cell lymphoma (typically the marginal zone form) and present as persistent, hard salivary gland swelling (**336**). Gamma-lineolic acid (oil of evening primrose) has been reported to be of help to patients with Sjögren's syndrome. Patients should be informed of the existence of the Sjögren's Syndrome Association and the Lupus Group, which are patient-led groups that provide support and help for sufferers.

Table 11 Features of special investigations in Sjögren's syndrome (SS)	
Stimulated parotid salivary flow rate	<0.5 ml/min
Labial gland biopsy	Focal lymphocytic infiltrate Duct dilatation Acinar loss Periductal fibrosis
Sialography	Sialectasis in parotid gland
Immunologic markers	
Rheumatoid factor	Positive in: 50% primary SS 90% secondary SS
Salivary duct antibody	Positive in: 10–40% primary SS 70% secondary SS
Anti-Ro (SS-A/SjD)	Positive in: 10% primary SS 65% secondary SS
Anti-La (SS-B/SjT)	Positive in: 60% primary SS 5% secondary SS

332 Ulnar deviation and swan neck deformities of the hands due to rheumatoid arthritis.

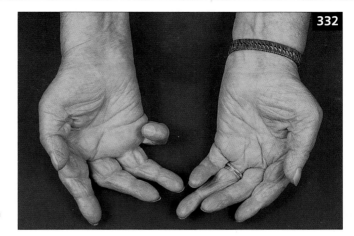

333 Facial 'butterfly rash' of systemic lupus erythematosus.

334 Bilateral parotid swelling in Sjögren's syndrome.

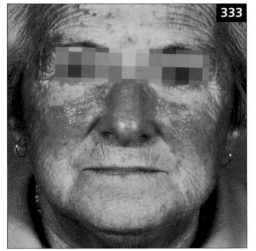

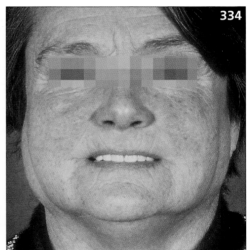

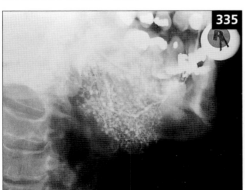

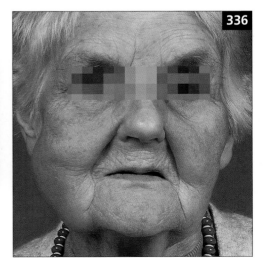

335 Parotid sialogram showing 'snow storm' punctate sialectasis.

336 Swelling of the right parotid gland due to lymphoma in a patient with Sjögren's syndrome.

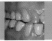

CREST syndrome

ETIOLOGY AND PATHOGENESIS
This condition is a variant of systemic sclerosis although the etiology is unknown.

CLINICAL FEATURES
Patients with this syndrome may present with an initial complaint of dry mouth. The particular features that provide the name CREST comprise subcutaneous **C**alcinosis, **R**aynaud's phenomenon, **E**sophageal dysfunction, **S**clerodactyly, and **T**elangiectasia.

DIAGNOSIS
No specific tests are yet available, although the presence of a range of auto-antibody markers are being explored. Diagnosis is usually achieved on the basis of the clinical features.

MANAGEMENT
Oral manifestations are managed as for any patient with xerostomia (pp. 166–167). Specific treatment for the underlying condition may involve the use of immunosuppressive agents or plasmaphoresis.

Excess salivation (sialorrhea)

ETIOLOGY AND PATHOGENESIS
Baseline production of saliva is often increased in a patient who has oral ulceration or is wearing a new denture for the first time. In such circumstances, stimulation of the salivary glands resolves once the ulceration heals or the oral tissues adapt to the new denture. Certain neuromuscular disorders, in particular Parkinson's disease and cerebral palsy, limit the ability to swallow and can result in apparent excess saliva.

CLINICAL FEATURES
There may be obvious pooling of saliva in the floor of the mouth (**337**) and drooling. However, it is not uncommon for patients to complain of excessive salivation but no clinical abnormality is present.

DIAGNOSIS
There are no specific tests to confirm the presence of excess salivation. The diagnosis is made on clinical observation alone.

MANAGEMENT
Surgical redirection of excretory ducts of the major salivary glands into the posterior oropharynx can be provided to patients with sialorrhea. A psychological assessment should be arranged for patients who have a complaint of excess salivation but clinical examination fails to reveal evidence to support this situation.

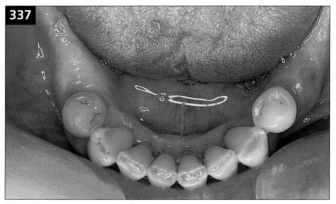

337 Saliva pooling in the floor of the mouth.

Coated tongue

ETIOLOGY AND PATHOGENESIS
The tongue has a natural coating in health due to the exfoliation of surface epithelial cells. However, failure of cells to be shed can lead to a surface layer (furring) that can produce a white or discolored appearance to the tongue. Coated tongue is a relatively frequent finding in patients with febrile illnesses or patients with a soft diet.

CLINICAL FEATURES
The coating on the tongue can vary in color from white through orange to brown, depending on external factors such as smoking or tea/coffee drinking (**338, 339**). Xerostomia may predispose to coating on the tongue (**340**).

DIAGNOSIS
Diagnosis is made on the basis of the clinical appearance.

MANAGEMENT
The patient should be reassured of the absence of any serious illness. Tongue hygiene involving gentle brushing of the tongue is helpful.

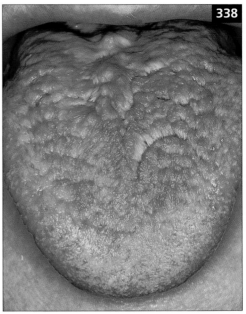

338 Elongation of the papillae on the tongue produces an appearance like hair, which can then become pigmented (brown or black hairy tongue).

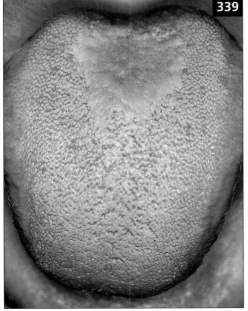

339 Coating of tongue in a patient who smoked.

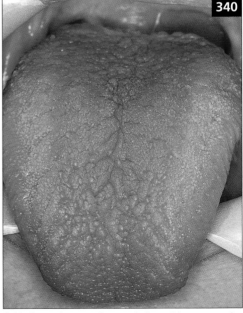

340 Coated tongue in association with xerostomia.

Halitosis (bad breath)

ETIOLOGY AND PATHOGENESIS

Poor oral hygiene or the presence of infection within the mouth is by the far the most frequent cause of halitosis. Odor develops due to the production of volatile sulfur (sulphur) compounds by oral bacteria, especially strict anaerobes. A marked or unpleasant smell also occurs in dehydration, renal failure, respiratory tract infection, cirrhosis, or diabetic ketosis.

CLINICAL FEATURES

Patients will complain that either they themselves or others have noticed the presence of bad breath. Obvious poor oral hygiene may be present (**341, 342**). However, it is not unusual for a patient complaining of halitosis to have good oral hygiene and no obvious problem. This has been referred to as delusional halitosis.

DIAGNOSIS

Halitosis can usually be detected by the simple smelling of exhaled breath. However, instruments for use in the clinic are available that measure volatile sulfur (sulphur) compounds within the breath and these may be helpful.

MANAGEMENT

Treatment should identify any local cause and underlying systemic disease. A good level of oral hygiene, including inter-proximal cleaning, should be achieved in all patients. Use of mouthwashes based on chlorhexidine, sodium bicarbonate, hydrogen peroxide, or sodium perborate may be helpful. Alcohol-based mouthwashes dry the mucosa and their use should be discouraged. Reassurance is all that can be given in the case of delusional halitosis.

Altered taste

ETIOLOGY AND PATHOGENESIS

Disturbance of taste can be caused by a number of disorders. Local factors include upper respiratory tract infection, xerostomia, smoking, radiotherapy, and medications. Neurologic disease, involving damage to the lingual nerve, chorda tympani, or facial nerve, or the presence of an intra-cranial tumor can result in the alteration or loss of taste.

CLINICAL FEATURES

The tongue and oral tissues usually appear healthy and the sole symptom is loss of taste. Occasionally, the patient may also complain of loss of smell since these two sensations are closely related.

DIAGNOSIS

Taste may be tested by the application of substances, such as salt, sugar, or lemon onto the dorsum of the tongue.

MANAGEMENT

Zinc, in the form of a mouthwash prepared from a 125 mg zinc sulfate (sulphate) tablet dissolved in water, has been suggested to be of some help. The mouthwash should be held in the mouth for 2 minutes three times daily.

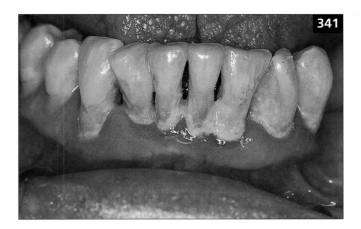

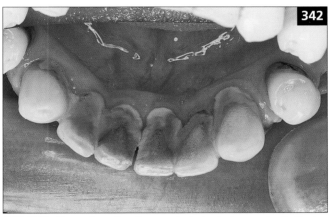

341, 342 Gross deposits of supra-gingival calculus causing halitosis.

Index